Holistic Dentistry.
Your Teeth. Your Body. The Correlations.

Dr. Stefanie Morlok

Dr. Stefanie Morlok:
Holistic Dentistry.
Your Teeth. Your Body. The Correlations
Bibliographic information published by Deutsche Nationalbibliothek:
The Deutsche Nationalbibliothek lists this publication in the Deutsche
Nationalbibliografie; detailed bibliographic data are available in the
Internet at www.dnb.de

morlok-books.de

ISBN 978-3-9818508-0-2
© First edition 2017

Author: Stefanie Morlok
First published in German under the title "Ganzheitliche Zahnmedizin –
Deine Zähne, Dein Körper, die Zusammenhänge" in 2015
Design & Cover design: Alois Gmeiner
Cover photo: zukhrufeya / fotolia.com
Cover back side photo: Dr. Stefanie Morlok
Pictures: see list of sources p. 122

Verlag: **morlok-books.de**

Contents

FOREWORD

From a young age, I was interested in a breadth of medical fields and treatments. Coming from a medical background, from the age of six years I already took great interest in the old medical books and the medical dictionary belonging to my grandfather. The body with all its interlinking facets has always exerted a great fascination upon me. One particular book of interest from my grandfather was a volume which dealt with the medical treatment of the oral cavity and its effects on the entire body.

Soon it was clear to me – I wanted to be a dentist. This subject promised to be very comprehensive and interesting. My family initially disliked the idea, they felt I should preferably study "proper medicine". Despite this, I thought from the beginning I would like to deal with medical practice via the mouth. I have now been practicing dentistry for almost 30 years and my initial calling has been a repeatedly satisfying experience. The mouth and its surrounding anatomy hosts a third of all body nerves – should this be the reason why the oral area seems to have such an incredibly large effect on the rest of the body?

Five letters with a significant meaning: the mouth

We speak, kiss, laugh, eat, drink, swallow and love with our mouths. We also taste with it and express our feelings with it. Quite a lot of functions for such a small body part. People are often oblivious to the fact that the direct and surrounding area of the mouth perform many more tasks than one thinks. An efficient functioning and well aligned oral area is important for the correct head position and is responsible for good breathing. The human mouth is unique. No other mammal has a similar mouth. We have unique teeth and a unique jaw. The human mouth is a tribute to the fact that we walk upright and on two legs. Without this it would not be the human mouth. The mouth has played an important role in the development of the human race.

An infant is born without teeth and without a significant oral cavity. By sucking on a mother's breasts, a baby builds its strength up, this supports the growth inside the mouth. The muscles of the lips, the tongue and the cheeks are strengthened. A vacuum that is produced during swallowing encourages the development of the teeth and the growth of the oral cavity. Oral diseases can affect many areas throughout the body.

A misalignment of teeth can prevent a proper bite. This can lead to stomach and further intestinal problems. An incorrect bite can cause problematic respiration, this occurs for example whilst breathing through the mouth. Respiration directly through the mouth causes throat inflammation and posture disorders.

A dead tooth or dental focus can damage the immune system. Diseased gums are discussed as a possible cause for heart and circulatory diseases. Badly aligned teeth can interfere with the posture and the development of the skeleton. And, and, and – the list of cause and effect is long and complicated. These numerous correlations play a decisive role in the field of holistic dentistry. The aim of this book is to give an overview of where, how and why.

Dr. Stefanie Morlok, summer 2015

For Heiko,
who always supported me in the realisation of this book.

Cause and effect:
Not many people know how to influence the causes.
They lose their times in trying to deal with the effects.

(Peter Hohl, Journalist)

1 DENTISTRY– A SHORT INTRODUCTION

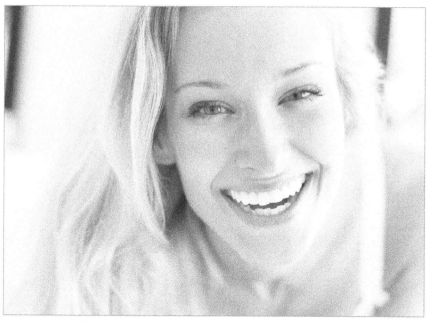

Fig. 1: Holistic dentistry looks at the tooth and the person attached to it.

1.1 From barbers, tooth pullers and dentists – a brief history.

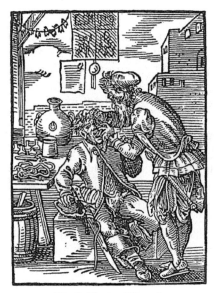

Fig. 2: The toothbreaker in the middle ages.

In earlier times, the treatment of teeth was not done by doctors. The barber as well as travellers were usually the ones to deal with aching teeth. In the Middle Ages they were called tooth crusher or – puller. It was not until the first quarter of the 18th Century that Friedrich Wilhelm, the First King of Prussia, stated in his medical reform from 1725 that the official German term of tooth doctor was to be used. Nevertheless, up until 1920 the barber surgeons were still operating.

According to the German "Reichsgewerbeordnung" from 1869, everybody could practice as a dentist. It is only since 1920 that dentists in Germany have been required to obtain an officially recognised qualification.

The course of dental history lead to dentistry being an entirely separate field of study from that of standard human medicine. Due to this, doctors are not trained in the area of dentistry and dentists only touch upon the basics of human medical practice.

Unfortunately, as a result, the connection between the diseased tooth or jaw joint and the rest of the body is to this day often dismissed as humbug or trivialized. Holistic dentistry is often associated with esoteric or dubious-treatment. This is a false impression and often the result of ignorance and uninformed opinion.

Exactly the opposite is important and correct: Dentistry must be seen and practised holistically.

1.2 The whole is better than a small part: Holistic dentistry looks at the tooth and the person attached to it

Holistic dentistry does not deal with only the teeth or the mouth, but takes the correlations of the body into account and hence chooses the adequate therapy. Dentistry always was a highly underrated area in the field of medicine. The term "dental plumber" says it all. The "proper" doctor put ones nose up when it came to dental treatment. The teeth and mouth are an extremely important part of the body. Without it not much can be done.

The teeth and their surrounding anatomy are part of the whole body. The health of this area is vital for our well-being. It is needed to eat, speak, laugh, swallow and it helps us to keep a good posture. The absence of teeth can cause damage to the cervical spine. If the jaw is affected by a dental focus or an inflammation, it may lead to general diseases.

Another important aspect of holistic dentistry is "how" dental treatment is implemented; it is important not to ask too much of a patient during treatment. The time of treatment is also a very important factor.

It is important to consider whether to perform the necessary treatment in the morning, the afternoon or in the evening; this differs from person to person. It is also important to consider the general well being of the patient on the day. Another interesting factor to take into account is which season of the year is suited best to the intervention as well as the most adequate lunar phase.

The bite should not be temporarily removed from the patient. The removal of toxins from the mouth may be channelled. The body should be strengthened before a detoxination. Dental materials must be chosen wisely, according to the requirements of the dental work, but also to the tolerance of the patient.

Empathy and consideration for the need, hardships and fears of patients is an important prerequisite for effective treatment. The individual need of each patient must be considered. What type of person a patient is and their constitution are of the utmost importance. All these aspects are part of holistic dentistry.

2 IT IS NOT JUST ABOUT A TOOTH: ALL THAT IS PART OF IT – THE CRANIOMANDIBULAR SYSTEM

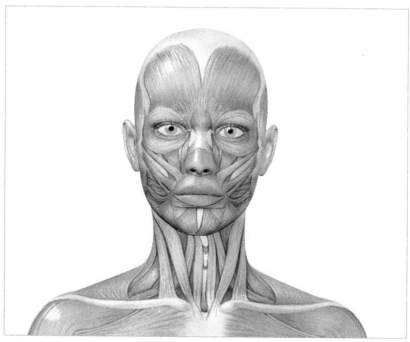

Fig. 3: The craniomandibular system does not only include the mouth but the entire head with the neck and the shoulder belt.

In holistic dentistry the tooth is not seen as a single entity by itself but in relation to the rest of the body. To get an impression of the complexity, in the picture below one can see an overview of the whole as a system with overarching cause-effect principles.

The craniomandibular system is the unit of teeth, tooth-bearing bones, jaws, jaw- and head joints, the cervical spine, all muscles surrounding the mouth, palate, the pharynx and all its nerves, blood vessels, lymphatic vessels and tissue. It includes the masticatory apparatus, the head, the neck, and upper shoulder area.

2.1   The basis: The tooth

You'll have to imagine the tooth as an onion. The outer layer is the enamel. It is the hardest substance in the human body and consists of calcium phosphate. The nest layer is dentinal; it consists of minerals, proteins and water. Those two hard layers surround the dental pulp. Herein are blood vessels, nerves and lymph vessels together in one channel. From the pulp, thousands of nerves radiate into the dentine. That is the reason why dentine is a living substance as opposed to enamel.

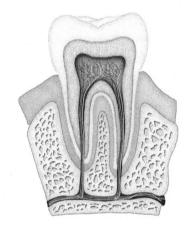

Fig. 4: The tooth and its anatomy.

Teeth are rooted in bone (periodontium). These roots are covered with a periodontal ligament. Below that is the root cementum, which in turn surrounds the pulp. Each tooth is attached via fine fibres into the jawbone. The gap where the ligament and the fibres are situated, is called the periodontal ligament. It is also equipped with nerves and blood vessels. All this is called the periodontal apparatus.

2.2   The tooth within the craniomandibular system

Healthy teeth are important. They are important for our diet: We need them to break up our food, to move it around in our mouth and to finally mix it with saliva. They play an important part in our appearance. A smile without teeth makes one look old. Only a baby can afford a toothless smile. Attractiveness has a lot to do with beautiful evenly placed and healthy teeth.

Healthy teeth are also important for other functions. To swallow in a healthy manner is only possible when teeth are in an optimum condition. A good bite is a prerequisite for good head and body posture. The cervical spine also benefits from the teeth being healthy.

More than 90 percent of the population suffer from one or more diseases relating to the teeth or gum area. These include cavities and periodontitis.

We are born into this world without teeth and it is seldom that we leave the world with all our own teeth intact. During breastfeeding a vacuum is produced in the oral cavity which helps the growth of the teeth. Unfortunately, using bottles does not attain the same effect. If resorting to bottle-feeding it is important to keep the teat opening as small as possible and therefore forcing the infant to make an effort. This will afford the necessary suction.

Once a child's first teeth have surfaced, the toddler will end up with 20 baby teeth. Ten in the upper jaw and ten in the lower jaw. They divide the oral cavity into the inner and the outer area of the mouth. From the beginning, the complicated interaction of the lips, teeth and tongue through to chewing, swallowing and breathing to head posture are all brought into play. Already at this stage, milk teeth can show signs of grave misalignment and positioning, which is often perpetuated through to the permanent teeth.

Many deformities are genetic or favoured by a genetic predisposition. Genetic deformities of the teeth and jaw could be caused by a certain degree of degeneration.

There can be many reasons for the existence of deformities. Deformations may occur during pregnancy, and or birth can play a role. Metabolic diseases, psychological problems, an overly large whole in a milk feeding bottle, accidents and bad habits such as thumb sucking or dummies can all act as catalysts. Even a lack of exercise or paying too little attention can lead to misalignment.

From the age of 5 to 7 years children start to lose their first teeth. The first molars start to grow behind the row of milk teeth, than slowly all the milk teeth are replaced by permanent teeth.

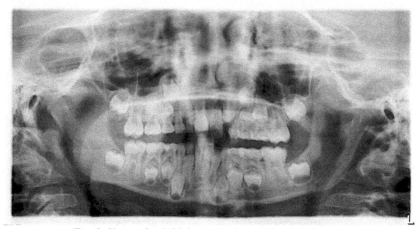

Fig. 5: X-ray of a child during teething – Panoramic view.

An adult person has normally 32 teeth altogether. The upper and lower jaw each contain 16 teeth.

The jaws are divided into four quadrants: the first and the second quadrant in the upper jaw, the third and the forth in the lower jaw. The teeth are numbered according to their position. Every quadrant holds 8 teeth; they are numbered from the middle outwards. The big incisor in front in the first quadrant is the "11". The first 1 refers to the quadrant and the second 1 for its position in the middle of the quadrant. It is pronounced one-one and not eleven. Children have a 5th and 6th quadrant in the upper jaw and a 7th and 8th in the lower jaw. The counting starts in the middle like in adult teeth.

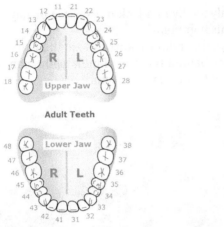

Adult Teeth

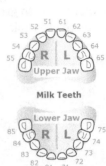

Milk Teeth

Fig. 6: Odontogram of an adult.   *Fig. 7: Odontogram of a child.*

The way the upper and lower jaw match each other is a miracle of nature. The curve of the upper jaw is slightly larger than the one of the lower jaw. This enables the lower teeth to interlock slightly with the upper teeth. Whilst biting, the teeth form two curves towards each other. One is the so called Spee curve, which goes from the front to the back, the other one is the Wilson curve which goes from the outside to the inside. Both curves allow for the teeth, jaws and muscles to function efficiently.

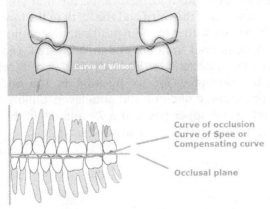

Fig. 8: Curves of the teeth to each other for maximum chewing efficiency.

The interlocking action is only possible due to the individual characteristics of each tooth. Every single tooth is equipped with cusps and ditches. The so called Fossa principle. The teeth of the upper and the lower jaws interlock. The bite of the two jaws is termed "occlusion".

The arch of the upper jaw is slightly wider than the arch of the lower jaw, hence the teeth of the upper jaw are situated on the outside in relation to the lower jaw.

2.3   The nerves in the craniomandibular system

The teeth of both jaws meet one another with a very fine point of contact with a barely perceptible sensitivity.

Think of a shotgun pellet which accidentally gets lodged between your teeth whilst eating a stewed rabbit. Even before consciously thinking "I've bitten on a piece of shot," the jaw immediately stops chewing to avoid greater damage. This is due to innervation – an area supplied by a high density of nerves. Such an area of nerves are to be found within the masticatory muscles of the jaw and the extremely sensitive nerves within the teeth.

A quarter of all body nerves are located within the area of the mouth and the jaw. In addition a

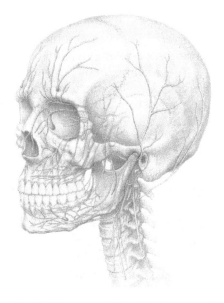

Fig. 9: The course of the facial nerve and the masticatory system.

third of all nerves run next to the jaw via the cervical spine into the body. For this reason the region of the teeth and the jaw joints are highly sensitive. If there is a problem with the bite, the joint of the jaw or the posture of the head, the results can have far reaching physical effects and disturbances.

The jaw has two nervous systems: the central nerve of each tooth and the nerve to the tooth socket (alveoli) of each tooth. The central nerve of each tooth is an extension of the trigeminal nerve. The trigeminal nerve is the third Cranial nerve. It supplies the individual teeth of both the lower and upper jaw.

Every tooth sits in a socket in the jawbone. The tooth socket is supplied by different nerves again.

When a bite is incorrect all anatomical structures in this area are affected. Also the nerves, which are usually in pairs are subject to unfavourable changes. The skull is a hub where nerves of the brain, the spinal cord and autonomic nervous system stem from, which through an incorrect posture of the head can all be compromised. The nerves within the jaw can be placed under too much stress through an incorrect bite. Even in joint of the jaw there is a high density of nerve fibre, the so called sympathetic nervous system.

These sympathetic nerve fibres are a related part of the autonomic nervous system, which can cause an organism to be stimulated. When damage occurs, this can result in an increased amount of nervous activity.

2.4 The jaws in the craniomandibular system

A big part of the facial skeleton is formed by the jaws. The upper jaw is part of the skull. The lower jaw occupies a special position. On the one hand it is connected to the skull via the mandibular joint, on the other hand it is part of the torso, since it is connected with the lower tongue and the muscles of the throat. The lower jaw moves toward the upper jaw to perform chewing, swallowing and speech functions.

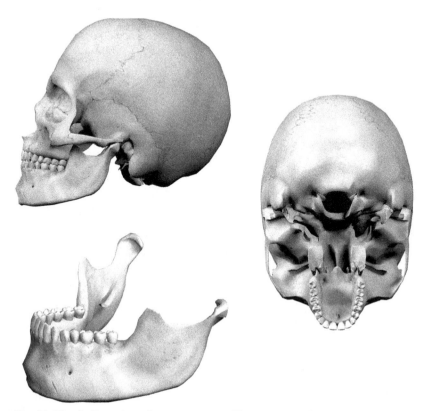

Fig. 10: The skull consists of two components, The cranium with the upper jaw and the independent bone of the lower jaw, which is also connected to the muscles of the chest.

2.5   The mandibular joint in the craniomandibular system

The mandibular joint is double headed joint, these are part of the lower jaw, the mandibular. They are placed in the so called "Fossa Mandibularis", within the temporal bone in the base of the skull. It can be felt, putting the little finger in one's ear and applying slight pressure. Now, open and close your mouth. Hereby you can feel the head of the joint of the lower jaw. Often you can also feel the articular disc gliding in between. The joint socket or mandibular joint is situated in the temporal bone, one joint being placed on each side of the skull. The so called temporomandibular-joint, the jaw joint is the most complicated joint in the body.

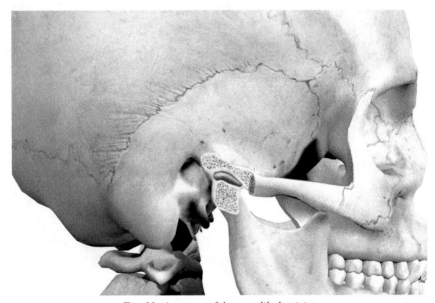

Fig. 11: Anatomy of the mandibular joint.

It is the only joint which has to function on both sides of the body in unison. This alone complicates the whole joint mechanism. The right and the left joint are separate entities, which are joined via the lower jaw allowing for a simultaneous operation. Therefore the mandibular joints can be compared to Siamese twins, which rely on each other to undertake effective movement.

In addition to this, the joint has to execute two movements in order for it to open the mouth. If you open your mouth slightly, the joint head rotates on its axis. If one opens the mouth wide, the joint head moves forward and out from the Fossa Mandibularis. This is known as first rotation and then translation. Condyloid joints – e.g. the wrist joint. Translation joints or facet joints – spinal joints.

Only the mandibular joint can do both. They rotate and slide. This is necessary for the movements of the jaw joints, like e.g. to open, to close and to move from back to front and to both sides. They are needed for chewing, for talking, for laughing, for swallowing, for singing and for stabilising and balancing the head on the cervical spine.

The mandibular joint is the only joint of the body which is controlled by a different part of the body, the teeth. They are not an active part of the joint, nevertheless they have to fit perfectly between the upper and lower jaw, to enable a smooth operational sequence.

Between the mandibular joints is a robust piece of cartilage, which saves the bones from rubbing on each other. The movement of the so called "articular disk" is very complicated. A small muscle, the upper part of the M. ptery-goideus lateralis is attached to the front of the articular disk. It pulls the disk forward if the mouth is opened. Attached to the back of the disk are elastic ligaments, which pull the disk back again if the mouth is closed.

During movement, the disk normally always sits on top of the head of the lower jaw. If there is a bite or joint malfunction or muscle tension the disk slides to the side or to the front, but it is seldom that it will moves backward. This will tend to increases problems in the joint.

2.6　The masseter muscles within the craniomandibular system

The skull is placed like a sphere on top of the cervical spine. The cervical spine is joined via the muscles with the shoulder. The mandible is joined via the muscles to the skull and via the hyoid bone to the sternum and the clavicles. Underneath the skull, a little bit behind the cervical spine, the neck and spinal muscles are attached. This complex muscle arrangement balances the head on the cervical spine.

To guarantee an effective function of all the actions of chewing, a perfect interaction of all these muscles is necessary.

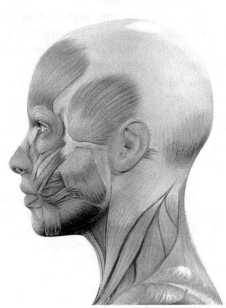

Fig. 12: Muscles of the head, the masticator apparatus and the neck.

If one could see into the skull from behind, the attachment of muscle would be clearly visible. The muscles of the skull are placed in such a way, so as to keep the lower jaw in relation to the upper jaw on a basis of permanent standby. The lower jaw should never be completely in permanent contact with the upper jaw because this would be far too strenuous for the teeth, the joints and the muscles. In a resting position the lower jaw should be slightly separated from the upper jaw, circa, 1-2 mm. Only whilst swallowing is it healthy to apply pressure between the two rows of teeth, one on top of the other.

It is called parking muscle, because it leaves the lower jaw awaiting its masticatory function. One can imagine here, that it's easy for light mistakes creep in. The consequence of an inaccurate bite is that the muscles are no longer symmetrical and of an uneven length, leading to tension due to a failure to keep the masticatory apparatus straight.

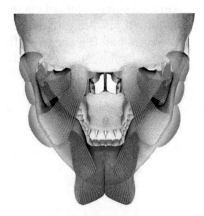

Fig. 13: The voluntary muscles of the jaw are influenced by the bite function.

2.7   The role of the head joints and the cervical spine in the craniomandibular system

The teeth, their bite, the jaw joints and the masticatory muscles are connected statically and dynamically to the cervical spine and the head joints. That means that a good bite is a prerequisite for a balanced cervical spine. If the bite is not straight, the temporomandibular joints are being stressed in an incorrect manner, the masticatory muscles are working lopsided and the result is an asymmetrical pressure and pull, also in the area of the neck and this therefore affects the cervical spine. An asymmetrical bite can also affect the shoulder. Far reaching problems can occur throughout the body and it is not seldom that this can even go down to the feet.

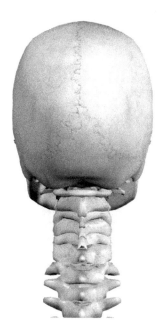

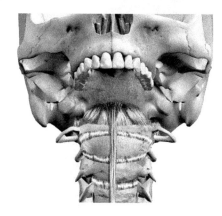

Fig. 14: The head joints, first cervical vertebra atlas with second cervical vertebra axis, both are joined via ligaments.

2.8 Lips, palate and tongue in the craniomandibular system

The form and fullness of the lips depends on the position of the jaw. Aesthetic dentistry puts a focus on how the lips are being highlighted through new dentures or a filling.

Well functioning lips are also important. The closure of the lips is a prerequisite for correct breathing and good mouth function. When breathing through the nose, caries and gingival inflammation is not contracted so easily, because the mouth does not dry out.

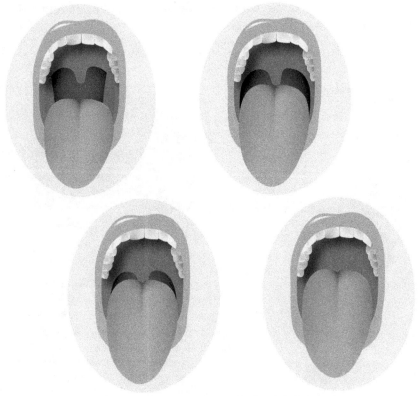

Fig. 15: The tongue, the palate and the lips.

A well developed palate is not too high, it is also broad and flat. We distinguish between a hard and a soft palate. We distinguish between a hard and a soft palate. The bone of the upper jaw is underneath the mucus membrane of the hard palate, the soft palate is behind the upper jaw in the throat.

Whilst swallowing, the tongue needs to be pressed onto the palate, and therefore the form of the palate is important for ones health. The palate is also important to move food around.

During this process, the food is also pressed with the tongue onto the palate in order to enable the throat to move it further. A palate which is too high or too flat can lead to problems in swallowing.

The tongue has many functions. It tastes food, whilst chewing, it moves food around the mouth, it is necessary for speech, it stabilises the head in its position, it is indispensable for swallowing and last but not least it is important for breathing.

2.9   The pharynx in the craniomandibular system

In alternative medicine, the pharynx is of uttermost importance, and its nature and position should always be assessed by the trained dentist. If there is little space in the pharynx, the patient has more of a gag reflex, which can be a hindrance during treatment and which is also a problem for the patient. Furthermore, a patient with a small pharynx is always susceptible to snoring or suffering breathing problems during the night. Patients with a deep bite or a back bite usually have a narrow pharynx, a problem which can be solved via orthodontics or bite raising.

The x-ray pictures of the lateral profile, the so called lateral cephalogram shows, that the diameter of the pharynx, known as the "upper airway space", is kinked differently and sometimes narrower, sometimes wider.

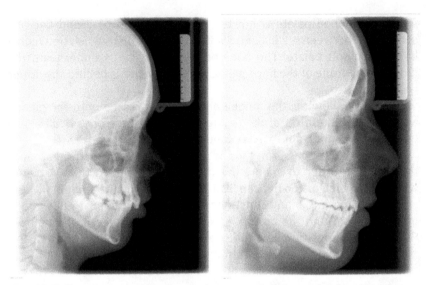

Fig. 16: Differently sized airway (upper airway space) during occlusal position change.

3 TREATMENT THROUGH HOLISTIC DENTISTRY – WHY AND WHERE DOES IT COME FROM?

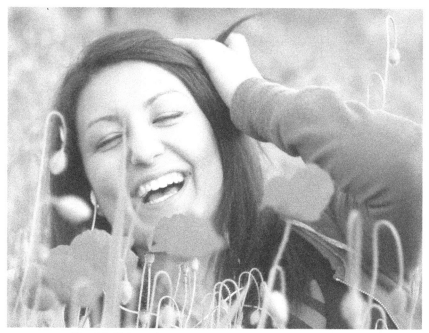

Fig. 17: Holistic dentistry is complex and finely coordinated.

3. TREATMENT THROUGH HOLISTIC DENTISTRY – WHY AND WHERE DOES IT COME FROM?

The system of the teeth, the mouth and the jaw with everything which is part of it is so complex and finely coordinated, that its balance can easily be upset. Holistic dentistry does not only see the illness by itself but relates it to the whole body. Thus, a detailed diagnosis is necessary with an according therapy, often requiring interdisciplinary treatments. The different treatments therefore have to engage with each other and depend on each other.

3.1 Classical and holistic: Different treatments in dentistry

3.1.1 Dentistry which is aimed to preserve for tooth decay and nerve inflammations

Tooth decay is one of the main illnesses of the teeth. Tooth decay means rotting teeth. Bacteria cause a softening of the enamel, the dentin, and/or the cement and with their acid excretion they soften the tooth substance and eventually it becomes carious. The bacteria slowly make their way forwards. The tooth tissue is eventually irrevocably destroyed and needs to be removed to what is left of the healthy part of the tooth. This is the so called "drilling" when one is at the dentist. Only once all the caries have been removed, the defect in the tooth can be filled. If the caries have reached the nerve, the tooth needs to undergo root treatment. In very severe cases the tooth has been destroyed by caries and needs to be removed. Caries can cause toothache. It is different with each individual at what stage caries causes tooth ache. If caries are not removed it can destroy a tooth.

Caries can be caused by consuming the wrong type of food. Especially white sugar and white flour can be held responsible for a change in the mouth flora, which then favours bacteria which cause caries. These and also drinks and foods containing sugar and also other sweeteners can contribute to causing caries. Sticky food is worse than food which runs down easily. The bacteria together with bits of food form a tough white layer – called plaque. It is the cause for the first little wound on the outside of the enamel, and it makes way for the bacteria to form caries.

When the oral flora changes and favours bacteria which are the cause for caries and periodontitis, the result is an acidic milieu in the oral cavity. The bacteria emit acids and also tissue-degrading enzymes which again are partly responsible for gum diseases. Once the bacteria have succeeded in producing a hole in the tooth or a gingival pocket underneath the gums, they find the ideal environment, without oxygen supply. This is the so called "anaerobic climate". In an anaerobic climate the bacteria thrive even better, and caries and periodontitis can flourish.

Due to the bacterial growth after consuming sugary foods, it is extremely important to have good mouth and dental hygiene. Especially in the gaps between teeth, it is very important to remove all the bits of food as well as plaque (an accumulation of concatenated bacteria which form a white tough layer). It is necessary to clean the teeth twice a day, namely in the morning and in the evening.

Another, not well known cause for oral diseases is the wrong respiration. A lot of people don't breathe through their nose but their mouths. The so called breathing through ones mouth. Breathing through the mouth can be the cause for many problems. The result can be pharyngitis, the development of poor posture and acidosis throughout the whole body. Inhalation through the mouth can be responsible for mouth acidosis. It is possible that this causes the area around the mouth and especially the teeth to dry out, which in turn fosters caries and periodontitis. Acidosis favours bacteria which cause caries and therefore the formation of caries itself.

The psyche and negative stress are also discussed as a possible causes for the development of caries and periodontal diseases. Presumably a weakening of the immune system has something to do with it. Hormonal problems, which are also seen as a possible cause, probably have the same interrelations.

Caries, incorrect pressure or metabolic problems can cause an inflammation of the nerve within the tooth. This results an inflammation of all the structures of the tooth nerve with its tissue in the nerve channel. The outcome is a higher circulation in this area, which causes unbearable tooth ache. This can only be relieved by opening the tooth. Subsequently the nerve of the tooth ends up being destroyed and the root canal is filled to avoid any further inflammations caused by bacteria.

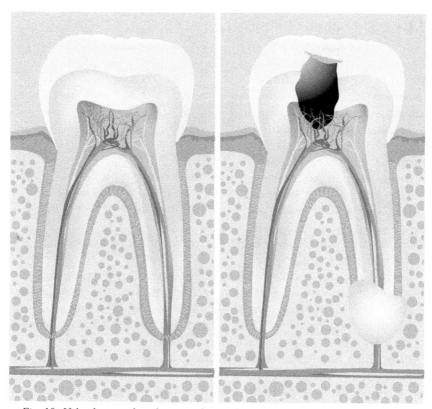

Fig. 18: If the damage done by caries has such an extent, that the nerve dies, a root filling is necessary.

When caries have caused defects or a loss of teeth, it should be repaired and every effort should be made to establish the former mouth situation with fillings or dentures. Aesthetic dentistry lends itself to be combined with holistic dentistry. I offer an array of options for aesthetic dentistry.

A perfect aesthetic result can be obtained and the transition between the tooth and the filling appear invisible. The natural tooth has a nucleus, the so called dentin, which is covered by the more transparent enamel. It can be reproduced with plastic or ceramic and no difference can be seen.

3.1.1.1   Aesthetic fillings

There is a German saying: "A smile is the most beautiful language in the world." Language appears even more appealing in combination with a beautiful smile. Aesthetic dentistry helps to provide harmonious looking teeth. This entails a nice colour, attractive teeth, a balanced array of the teeth in

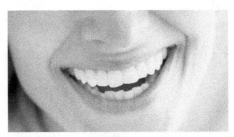

Fig. 19: A perfect result can be achieved with a high quality filling for the front teeth.

relation to the jaw. The lips and the surrounding soft tissue are also taken into consideration.

If caries has formed and a filling is necessary, it is possible to fill the tooth in varying ways. When it comes to the incisors, the only option is a direct plastic filling or veneer (dental laminate). The fillings can be done with normal plastic. Under certain lighting conditions it will not always be possible to conceal these procedures.

The filling can also be done with a special plastic which imitates the optical appearance of the incisor. This means a special plastic is used for the inner filling and consequently different plastics are layered over it, all in the same colour, but with a different translucency. The appearance can also be changed by using different colours. Hereby a perfect aesthetic appearance can be achieved and no transition between tooth and filling can be seen. The natural tooth has also got a nucleus, the so called dentin, and it is covered by the more translucent enamel.

3.1.1.2   Ceramic inlays

The side teeth can be directly filled
with plastic. Though they are not as
durable as the qualitatively much
better insert fillings, the so called
inlays. When this method is used, first
all the caries are removed. The tooth
together with the dental defect are
prepared by making a surround to
make a form. An imprint is made and
the tooth is temporarily filled with a
plastic filling. After 1 to 2 weeks the
ceramic inlay which has been
fabricated in the laboratory is then
glued into the tooth. This ensures a
perfect fit and an aesthetically
pleasing result.

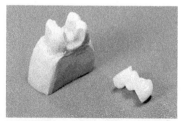
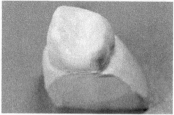

*Fig. 20: Preparation of a tooth for a
ceramic inlay.*

3.1.1.3   Crowns

If the teeth are severely damaged by caries or an accident, they have to
have a crown. Hereby the tooth is diminished in size, in order for the
crown to sit on top like a well fitting hat. The filed tooth is completely
covered with the crown and the gap between the crown and the tooth
has to be entirely sealed tight to ensure that caries can not get
underneath the crown.

Crowns can be made out of ceramic, gold, a conglomerate of metal
and ceramics, circonoxyd with or without ceramic or plastic. The
dentist chooses together with the patient, which material is the right
one. The cost, individual requirements, and aesthetic considerations
hereby play an important role. The tolerance of the material is of the
uttermost importance and should be tested individually.

On the basis of more and more radiation around us, nowadays the usage of metal in the mouth must be seen in a different context to former times. By considering meticulously the individual aesthetic wishes of the patient and thanks to the latest techniques, it is possible to insert crowns which look like natural teeth and hence bearing little resemblance to the appearance of crowns at all. Irregularities of the natural teeth can therefore be completely eliminated and a perfect, regular smile is the result.

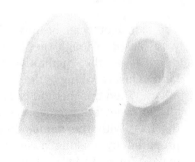

Fig. 21: Ceramic Crowns.

3.1.1.4   Veneers (Laminates)

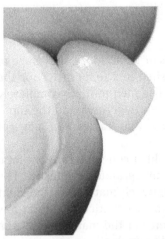

Fig. 22: Veneers decisively improve the aesthetic of the front teeth.

If teeth are not affected by caries but do suffer from other aesthetic problems, veneers should be taken into account. In some cases a patients tooth or teeth may not even need any form of preparation, whereby the tooth sustains injury. The veneer can be glued directly onto the area of the faulty host tooth which is visible and thus avoiding unnecessary dental work. The result is a perfect smile with a minimum effort.

3.1.2 Periodontitis – Periodontal disease

Gum diseases (Parodontopathien, Parodontitis) are as common as caries. People often refer to it as gum disease but the proper term is periodontitis. The tooth, the gums, the bone in which the tooth is imbedded and the fibres between the tooth and the bone form the periodontium, the whole "apparatus" which hold the tooth. Periodontitis means an inflammation of this whole "apparatus".

The first step before the onset of a periodontitis is a gingivitis – an inflammation of the gingivia, which is another term for the gums. A reddening and swelling is the result and if this is not cured in a short space of time, it spreads to the root skin of the tooth and the fibres and eventually to the whole surrounding bone. It reacts to the inflammation by shrinking. This means the bone starts to shrink and shorten, visibly exposing the neck of the tooth separating from the gum, which also recedes, together with the bone.

If periodontitis is not treated the loss of a tooth and even the bone can be the result.

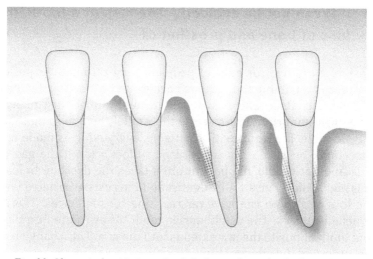

Fig. 23: If a periodontitis is not healed, the result can be the loss of tooth.

As it is the case for caries, bacteria are also responsible for periodontitis. A key role is the interaction of food, dental hygiene and the acid base balance. The metabolism and its supply with vitamins and trace elements is important, one can think of the illness of scurvy caused by a lack of vitamin c, a condition which made sailors lose their teeth. Hormonal deficiencies are nowadays under discussion as a possible cause for periodontitis.

In holistic dentistry, when treating peritonitis, the intestines are always treated simultaneously, because an intestinal imbalance can add to an imbalance in the mouth. The mouth is after all the beginning of the digestive tract. Immune illnesses and certain medicines can be an additional factor for peridotites or the trigger. A key aspect when it comes to cum diseases is an incorrect bite. When the bite is not correct, this can lead to stress and hence inflammation of the dental structure.

With gum diseases, a holistic prophylaxis is especially important, to prevent a reoccurrence of any inflammation. The deciding factor is, that all the contributory elements causing the inflammation are taken into account, so that in the future one knows what to avoid or improve.

3.1.3 If it can not be avoided – The loss of a tooth, the loss of bone and prosthetics

The loss of a tooth is for a lot of people a very traumatic experience. Often there is a painful and tedious background of tooth ache, painful treatments, etc. Once one has pulled through all of this, many are unaware how important it is to close the gap left by a missing tooth as soon as possible. If a front tooth is missing, every effort is made to find a replacement because ones appearance suffers a lot. If the gap is on the side and not visible, the patient often takes the decision to leave it like it is and avoids a visit to the dentist and the costs associated with it.

The loss of a tooth can have far reaching consequences. There are many disadvantages. The neighbouring teeth tilt or rotate into the gap and the tooth opposite the jaw extends into the gap. This change results in a negative and detrimental bite.

The teeth are put under undue stress, the consequence are gum and bone damage. Jaw joint problems develop as a result. Finally, this can lead to problems for the whole body, like posture problems and joint complaints. In addition, the bone might degrade where there is a missing tooth.

It is therefore wise to always consider an implant or a bridge in the event of losing a tooth, because the long term damage is often worse than the initial treatment and costs.

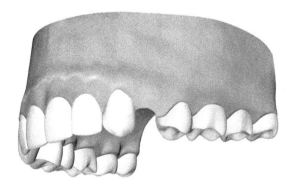

Fig. 24: If a gap in a row of teeth is not closed, the consequence for the bite and the masticatory apparatus are negative.

The degradation of the bone within the mouth can also have far reaching consequences for the patient. There are various reasons and causes for bone degradation around teeth:

1. Initially the tooth develops a caries which is then followed by a dental nerve inflammation. The resulting inflammation subsequently causes the decay of the nerve. The consequence of such an inflammation affects the tip of the root of the tooth, which then leads to a deterioration of the bone where the tooth is rooted.

2. Gingivitis, which can be caused by incorrect oral hygiene practices, can result in a gingival pocket and eventually in a gum bone pocket. More and more bacteria accumulate, which

then spread the inflammation further. A repercussion of this is an increased reduction of the bone mass and finally the tooth loosens and eventually falls out.

3. False contacts during the bite as well as overstraining can also cause the formation of gum bone pockets, which then can lead to the loss of a tooth.

4. Some general illnesses, for example diabetes, can lead to or foster gingivitis and a loss of bone.

5. If a tooth is lost, the bone in this area will eventually begin to deteriorate.

3.1.3.1 Dentures

There is a distinction between fixed and loose dentures. Thanks to implants, nowadays it is in most cases possible to have fixed dentures. This is dependent of course on the price one is prepared to pay and also the condition of the bone. If implants are too costly or if the existing bone is not sufficient enough and a restructuring of the bone would be very difficult or extremely costly, it would then be recommended to utilise standard dentures.

If there are no teeth at all, so called complete dentures are made. The manufacture and setting of these teeth provides a creative and therapeutically functional challenge. The combination of aesthetics, an efficient chewing function and the correct positioning of a prosthesis, is difficult task for both a dentist and dental technician. It is also necessary for a patient to have perseverance.

If only a few teeth are missing, partial dentures can be utilised. What distinguishes this sort of denture is the method of fastening. There are simple partial dentures, which fasten using metal brackets that attach to the remaining teeth either side of a gap. There are other, more complicated attachments or telescopes which cause less damage to teeth rather than brackets and which are optically more pleasing. Other refinements like mounting bolts can be included.

The materials used for normal dentures include metal for the frame, and acrylic for the gums, saddles and teeth. Nowadays injection moulding plastics can also be used for the frame of a prosthesis. Telescopes and attachments used to be made exclusively out of metal, but nowadays they can be made out of injection moulding plastics and also out of zirconium oxide. In this case, everything is white and "metal free", apart from the fact that zirconium as an element is considered a metal. The great advantage of metal free dentures is the much lighter weight of the reconstruction. Furthermore, zirconium oxide is non conductive and therefore negates the generation of harmful electrical currents in the mouth.

In some cases the dental situation can not be solved with a fixed denture. Therefore the only possibility is the use of non fixed dentures. One differentiates between complete dentures, if the patient has no teeth left in the jaw or partial dentures, if some teeth are left and the dentures can be fixed onto them. There are different forms of partial dentures. The simple version is equipped with bend or cast clips. The aesthetic result is not very pleasing and places more burden on the teeth than other alternative methods of fixing. Improvements have already been attained by using the new injection moulding plastic technology, due to the fact that the clips are made out of flexible plastic which matches the colour of the teeth. The big advantage of the injection moulding plastic technology is the fact that the plastic has only a tiny amount of monomers which renders the plastic less toxic. Injection moulding plastic is easier to polish and is subsequently smoother and therefore less bacteria are able to adhere to it.

The fasteners for partial dentures are called telescopes. A telescope consists of an inner and an outer crown, and together they are responsible for the support of the prosthesis. The inner crown is cemented onto the tooth, the outer crown is inside the prosthesis. The outer crown can be slid exactly onto the inner crown. Telescopes are a very aesthetically pleasing solution. The fastening of the prosthesis is invisible.

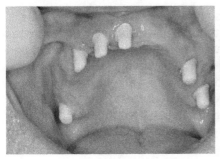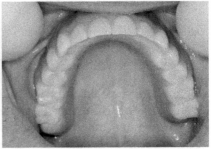

Fig. 25: With telescopes it is possible to invisibly fasten a prosthesis.

Another variation is the usage of so called "attachments". The remaining teeth are covered by crowns which have little pins or push-buttons on the side. The sockets for these pins or push-buttons are incorporated into the prosthesis and so they can be slid on or pressed on. The prosthesis remains anchored and no fasteners can be seen.

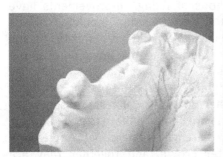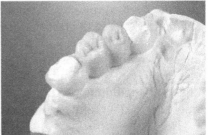

Fig. 26: With a partial mini denture manufactured using plastic injection moulding, a gap in the middle of the teeth or at the end can be dealt with without any problems.

A special variant of the partial denture is the partial mini denture. In this instance only a few teeth may be missing which for various reasons can not be replaced by a bridge. A partial mini denture can be made out of injection moulding plastic, which is then attached via discrete white ring clamps that are also removable. It cannot unfasten itself, because thanks to the flexibility of the plastic clamps a firm hold onto the teeth can be guaranteed.

3.1.3.2 Bridges

When single teeth are lost and implants are out of the question, a bridge is often the best solution.

There are several different forms to choose from. A bridge consists of two teeth, one on either side of a gap of which both are provided with a crown. The gap between the crowns are connected via a bridging structure. The bridge structure is a denture fitted to span the gap. A bridge can also be made out of partial crowns or fillings.

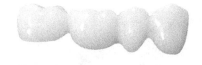

Fig. 27: With a bridge a gap in the teeth can be "bridged over".

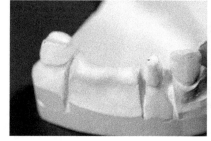
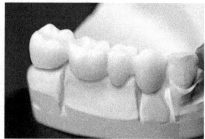

A special bridge is the Maryland bridge. The teeth providing the bridge abutments are not ground down, but are fitted with multifaceted stickers to keep the bridge structure in the gap.

Bridges can be cast out of metal, they can later be coated with ceramic and they can also be made out of zirconium oxide, with or without ceramic. With the new injection moulding plastics, durable bridges can also be made out of this material.

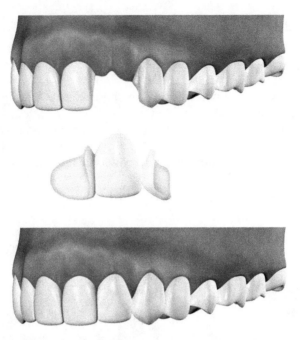

Fig. 28: The Maryland bridge consists of a non visible clip support which is stuck onto the teeth, and in between, it has an integrated bridge structure. This saves the teeth having to be ground.

3.1.3.3   Metal free dentures

Nowadays, innovative technologies have enabled the production of aesthetic dentures without the usage of metal. Patients suffering from allergies and who are susceptible to radiation can benefit from it.

Many constructions were only possible if made from metal. New technologies like zirconium oxide prosthetics and injection moulding plastics have made way for new possibilities. Fillings are not suitable if the defects are on a larger scale or if a tooth is lost. Dentures have to "whip everything back into shape."

Normally dentures are, at least partially, made out of metal. New methods enable the production of dentures for almost every situation without having to use metal.

Telescopic or attachment crowns can be made from zirconium oxide, prosthesis out of monomer free injection moulding plastics. Monomer is the poisonous element contained in conventional plastic.

Usually, even in difficult circumstances it is usually possible to find a solution without metal.

This makes it possible to produce dentures which are more aesthetically pleasing and also lighter.

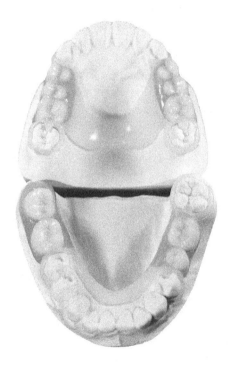

Fig. 29: With metal free dentures a greater degree of comfort is attainable.

3.1.3.4   Implants – or the art to make everything afresh

To have firmly fitting teeth up to a ripe age is nowadays no problem. Thanks to a sophisticated implant system and various options for bone replacements, firm fitting artificial teeth are possible for almost every patient.

Especially when using implants it is important to verify if the materials used are tolerated by the patient. It is also crucial to prepare the metabolism beforehand to ensure that the body accepts the foreign materials without any problems and that the healing is a smooth process. There can be further intolerances which can be dealt with easily.

Implants are often a better solution than a bridge, because the neighbouring teeth don't have to be ground. An implant is often a more aesthetic solution than a bridge.

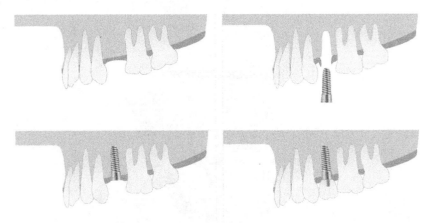

Fig. 30: Implants are artificial roots made out of titanium or zirconium oxide.

Methods of detoxification, the reinstallation of the acid-base balance and the administration of minerals which build up the bone are of uttermost importance before an implantation. Today, unfortunately there are lots of patients who take medication against osteoporosis, the so called bisphosphonates. The use of these medications is a strict contraindication against implants. Such patients are not able to benefit from implants because of the inability to be able to heal. Science has not yet found all the answers in this field.

It is suspected that due to the use of bisphosphonate a less efficient supply of bone is the consequence and this and could lead to an unsuccessful healing process when dealing with implants. Also other pharmaceuticals, e.g. chemotherapeutics can hinder the healing process following an implant.

There have been various forms of implants. The following such as plate implants, cylindrical implants and disc implants were commonplace. Until recently, screw implants have prevailed. There is a differentiation between implants which consist of one or several parts. Systems which consist of more than one part have a better prospect of healing successfully because they lay underneath the mucous membrane. As soon as the screw of the implant has healed, the upper parts can be screwed in. The advantage is, that during the healing process they do not stick out and it makes it impossible for any bacteria to get in via the open wound into the bone.

Alongside titanium implants, usage of ceramic implants were once widespread. Eventually though due to the risk of breakages, ceramic implants were all but abandoned. Titanium implants have remained the standard. Recently there has been the introduction of implants made from zirconium oxide, which are substantially problematic in the healing process. Allegedly though it is less responsible for material intolerance in comparison to titanium, but titanium is still an effectively compatible material.

As Titanium is a metal it is often rejected in naturopathic medicine. Zirconium oxide is often referred to as ceramic implant. This is not completely true, zirconium oxide is strictly speaking a metal oxide derived from zirconium. It is mined and then made into powder which is then sintered into a ceramic like form. Another reason as to why zirconium oxide is popular is because it is white and titanium is grey.

Dentures like crowns or bridges fixed to implants is a specialised procedure, using specific methods and parts. For it to be successful it crucial that the work is done precisely. The preparation of a tooth in a special form is then fitted with the relevant crown.

A healing screw or cover screw is removed from an implant with an inner threading, after surgically opening the implant. Then an abutment is screwed in and finally a crown is fitted exactly on top of it. Implants can be very useful as abutments for dentures or prosthesis, especially in cases when there only a minimal amount of teeth left in the jaw, implants are the only solution for a good fitting denture.

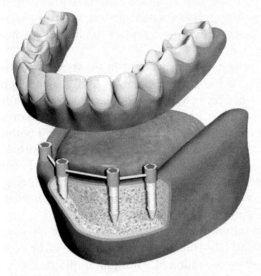

Fig. 31: Implants ensure a firm fit of dentures.

3.1.4 Dental Operation – Dental Surgery

A holistic approach is particularly important when having to resort to surgery. Surgery cannot always be avoided in dentistry. This includes the removal of decayed teeth, wisdom teeth, apicoectomy and gum operations. To achieve a more effective healing process it is useful to complement the dental treatment with holistic or natural healing methods. For instance the functional analysis of the bite and the mandibular joint, the search for the best time for the operation, the use of magnetic field therapy, bioresonance therapy, homeopathy and orthomolecular measures. Even taking into consideration the lunar phase or the time of the day can have positive effects on the course of treatment. It is of great importance to consider the individual metabolism, metabolic problems or other illnesses.

During operations, the patient is usually nervous. Therefore it is better to create a relaxed atmosphere in the surgery. A talk between the dentist and the patient might be a good idea. The treatment should occur in a quiet room. I work together with psychotherapists and hypnotists to prepare patients with fear issues pertaining to dental surgery before an operation. After an operation it is important for the patient not to be left with an unsightly gap or similar. They will be provided with a temporary replacement to hide the defect.

I observe and find it of particular importance to elicit the best moment during the lunar calendar. This is obviously only medically possible when the situation allows and not when the patient needs emergency treatment.

Surgical dental appointments should be made during a waning moon; During a waxing moon (the first quarter of the moon) and Taurus and Aries, surgical treatments are unfavourable.

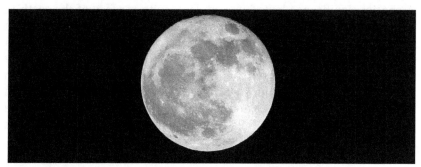

Fig. 32: When performing dental operations, consideration of the lunar calendar is important.

During a waning moon, one is less sensitive to pain. Wounds bleed less and is healing quicker.

When teeth are removed this causes scaring which may then cause some sort of interference. Through neural therapy, bio resonance therapy or isopathy (see chapter "good vibes"), these disturbances can be addressed.

51

3.1.4.1   Removal of wisdom teeth

Every effort is made to preserve wisdom teeth. After all, wisdom teeth have a correlation to the heart and the small intestine. Particularly in children and adolescents, effective orthodontic work makes more space available in the jaw bone. By the emergence of a wisdom tooth it is often a painful experience. It is possible to reduce this pain by resorting to a small operation accompanied by using medication, homeopathic treatment or alternative medicine. In some cases, unfortunately, the tooth can't be preserved. The rules for dental operations are the same as for the above described dental operations.

3.1.4.2   Apicoectomy

A special significance have infected roots with regards of the teeth in relation to organs. If the point of a root treated tooth gets infected afresh, and a bone infection is the result, an apicoectomy is often needed. This signifies, that an operation is necessary and that the tip of the tooth which suffers from the inflammation is being removed. Often a root treated tooth is a nidus which can affect the whole body. After an apicoectomy it should be tested in regular intervals, if the focus is still there. It can be tested via Electroacupuncture after Voll (EAV) or via kinseological tests. Even bloodtests can be helpful.

3.1.4.3   Dental focus- or the healing of bone infections

The tip of a root treated tooth can newly be infected. This can cause an infection which affects the whole body. Also the area of the jawbone from which the tooth has been taken out can be newly infected or not heal completely. This infection can cause problems throughout the whole body. A root treated tooth needs the removal of the old root filling and the making of a better new one.

   With regards to the jaw bone a surgical reconstruction of the bone is necessary, herby the bone is cleaned mechanically. This can be supported with natural healing methods. Dental focuses are held responsible for chronical illnesses throughout the body. For instance heart-, joint-, or kidney problems can be caused by a dental focus. Often these complaints finish after a the dental focus has been treated.

3.1.4.4   Periodontal Operations

If presented with a heavy periodontitis, sometimes a few teeth which have suffered an especially bad bone loss have to undergo small surgery. This is the only way to ensure no further reduction of the gums or even stimulate repairing growth. It is important to exclude that the cause lies within the hormones or the intestine. If problems are herein present illnesses of the gums are not rare. Also a too strong bite on a single tooth can cause gum problems with bone reduction and therefore a functionality and bite analysis is always indicated.

3.1.4.5   Bone formation

When implants or dentures are being made a solid amount of bone is necessary. If there is not enough bone, it needs to be rebuild. How to proceed here differs form case to case and is individually very different and needs to be defined individually for every case. After the bone has been rebuild one needs to wait for 4 to 6 months before further measures can be taken. Here the use of holistic methods is also possible.

3.2   Malocclusions

A normal bite is rare. Like it is described in the chapter "The teeth in the craniomandibular system" a normal or perfect dentition, has different criteria: The dental arches are formed harmonically, the teeth fit onto the alveolar ridge. The upper jaw is a bid wider than the lower jaw to enable the morsal surface to have an interlocking bite. The bite is not too deep and one front tooth is not too much above the other. The points of the canine teeth of the upper jaw protrude into the interdental space of the lower canine teeth and the small canine teeth which lies behind. The point of the cusp of the first big upper canine tooth protrudes into the middle groove of the lower first big canine tooth in front.

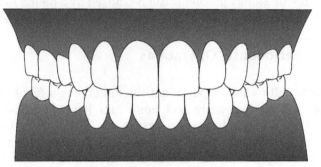

Fig. 33: Perfectly positioned teeth.

A lot more diffused are malpositions of the teeth which I want to show you on the following pages using tables.

3.2.1 Retrusive Occlusion

Retrusive occlusion means that the lower jaw is too far behind with regards to the upper jaw. Usually it is in combination with a compression of the mandibular joint and a forward head position.

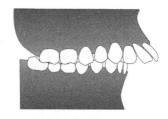

3.2.2 Overbite

When an overbite occurs, the lower jaw, in relation to the upper jaw, is too far forward. This is often combined with the tension of the cervical spine and a backward head position.

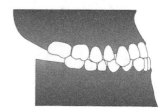

3.2.3 Open Bite

The open bite can be caused by a dysfunction of the tongue or the lip. This causes a gap between the upper and lower jaw front teeth. This is often combined with the patient breathing through the mouth and a compression onto the head joint. If the extension of the first cervical vertebrae reaches too far into the foramen magnum* the result might be a compression onto the brainstem.

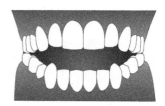

* The foramen magnum is the hole in the skull through which the spinal marrow extravagates.

3.2.4 Deep Occlusion

Deep occlusion means that the height of the teeth from top to bottom is altogether decreased. Responsible for this are often side teeth which fail to protrude properly out of the bone or which grow too shallow. When a deep bite is present, the mandibular joint is normally too clinched, this favours a forward position of the head.

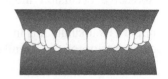

3.2.5 Crossbite

Crossbite means that the rows of teeth are positioned the wrong way round. That means that the upper jaw or a part of it is narrower than the lower jaw. We differentiate the complete crossbite when the whole upper jaw is smaller than the lower jaw, the two sided crossbite, when only the side are of the teeth of the upper jaw is too small, the one sided crossbite (see picture) when only one side of the upper jaw lies to much on the inside and the frontal crossbite, this occurs when the front teeth of the upper jaw lie behind the front teeth of the lower jaw without an overbite being present.

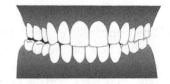

3.2.6 Cusp On Cusp Bite

When the upper jaw sits squarely over the lower jaw, this often results in the cusps or the peaks and edges of teeth resting directly on one another instead of being able to interlock. The same variations are possible as with the cross bite.

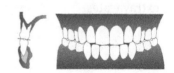

3.2.7 Non Occlusion

Non occlusion is a dysfunctional bite, whereby the operation and usage of the upper and lower jaws misaligns the teeth. There are the so called buccal (cheek-side) and lingual (tongue side) non occlusions.

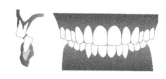

3.2.8 Crowded Teeth

Crowded teeth often occur due to a misalignment on the alveolar ridge. The cause for this is either there is not enough space on the alveolar ridge or that the teeth are too large.

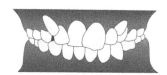

3.2.9 A Narrow Jaw

The upper and/or the lower jaw are too narrow and are not compatibly shaped.

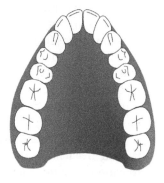

3.2.10 A Combination Of Malocclusions

All malocclusions can occur completely or partially. They can be combined with other malocclusions. It could therefore be that a patient has a deep bite with a retrusive occlusion and also crowded teeth.

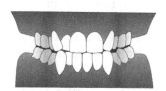

3.3 Consequences of misaligned teeth

Misaligned teeth are not only a cosmetic problem. The positions of teeth play an important part in having healthy teeth. If teeth are misaligned, illnesses relating to the teeth or the mouth are very probable. Even illnesses affecting the whole body can manifest themselves through having problems with teeth.

Misaligned teeth can cause a person to experience mild to severe health impediments. Some misalignments cause problems when closing the mouth properly which can in turn lead to further complications involving breathing and other respiratory difficulties. Breathing through the mouth fosters tooth decay and periodontitis. It is more problematic to clean crowded teeth and the stress on individual teeth causes imbalances, which again can lead to caries and bone reduction of the periodontal bone. A narrow jaw leaves too little space for the tongue and this can initiate speech problems.

The impairment of a tongue can also lead to problems in chewing and swallowing. In particular, breathing problems and associated problems caused by the tongue due to misaligned teeth, can mar the development of a child. One cannot underestimate the detrimental effects of a faulty bite in relation to the surface for chewing; this can foster neurological symptoms and problems with posture. An incorrect bite is often responsible for tooth ache, tooth fractures and periodontitis, which can eventually lead to the loss of a tooth.

Even headaches and problems with the mandibular joint can be caused by a faulty bite. Often these complaints are accompanied by tension to the head and facial muscles. Even if aesthetic considerations are often not seen as a medical necessity, I want to point out the psychological damage caused by severely misaligned teeth and the consequent disfiguration of an otherwise potentially attractive person. These are all reasons as to why orthodontics, which deal with all these problems, is an extremely important part of medicine and dentistry.

3.4 Orthodontics

"Back to health." The aim of orthodontics is to restore a patient's health, away from illness and dysfunctional teeth. Holistic orthodontics focuses particular attention to the function of the mouth and the masticatory apparatus. The aesthetic aspect – which is important and will correct itself alone with proper treatment – is secondary in the face of the functional task of orthodontics. It is of crucial importance, that after orthodontic treatment the bite is examined. If problems cannot be resolved with orthodontics alone, other additional therapeutic measures have to be taken.

3.4.1 Holistic Orthodontics

Conditions like a stooped posture, a forward head position, jaw pains, head, neck and facial pains as well as orthopaedic related pain and ear symptoms like tinnitus can be treated with holistic functional orthodontics. Not only children but adults can also benefit from holistic orthodontics. It improves the head posture, encourages breathing through the nose, enables one to close the lips properly, shapes the jaw line, enables proper swallowing, optimises the metabolism, loosens the tissue and the muscles, dissolves lymphatic blockages and even encourages skeletal regeneration.

3.4.2 Breathing through the mouth

A lot of children experience problems as the closure of the mouth develops, with nasal breathing and the correct positioning of the tongue. Breathing through the mouth is especially problematic for the development of the jaw and the position of the head and hence the whole body. Often with small children this is caused by weak muscle structure or the effects of a first cold, the effects of which remain.

When breathing through the mouth, the lung is only partially inflated and this leads a general over production of acids in the tissue. The mouth area becomes too cold, the teeth are dry out and defects through caries are more likely, especially for teeth at the front of the mouth. The paranasal sinuses don't get enough air and the result is, is the inadequate development of these bones and especially that of the upper jaw, whereby then the upper jaw is too small and therefore there is not enough space for the tongue.

This creates a vicious cycle. As the tongue grows bigger one is forced to breath through the nose. To be able to do this, the head needs to be held forward the teeth need to be pressed together to help the muscles, leading to deep bite and a reduced inner mouth area which is then too small. Holding the head forward encourages a narrowing of the throat tract and this can then encourage inflammations to occur such as tonsillitis.

This is a reason as to why children can be affected by sleep apnoea at an early age. During sleep they cannot inhale enough air or no air at all.

With adults it is also relevant if they breathe through the mouth or the nose. It seems to be beneficial to equip people, who persistently breathe through their mouth, with a Bionator, as a bite splint and to complement the treatment with speech and pronunciation therapy. It is particularly important to improve the mouth closure with myofunctional exercises.

3.4.3 Loose and fixed orthodontic appliances

In orthodontics one has to always make the decision as to whether to use a removable or fixed orthodontic appliance. In individual cases both forms might be necessary.

For small children, removable apparatus' are recommended. A fixed appliance usually only makes sense when all the remaining teeth have come through and when the improved orthodontic function is evident after the use of a removable device. Therefore it is extremely important to treat children as early as possible with removable appliances so as to positively influence the growth of the jaw, there are countless orthodontic appliances. The following are a few examples which have already proven to be successful:

3.4.3.1 Orthodontic Plates

Orthodontic plates are devices designed to fit the upper or lower jaw, which contain parts such as extendible screws or braces to move the teeth or the jaw area and stretch it.

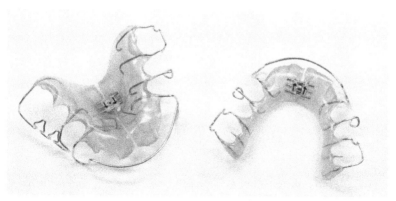

Fig. 34: Removable Orthodontic Plates.

3.4.3.2   Bionator

Already at the beginning of the last century devices for relaxing and improving the function of the mouth were developed by dental scientists.

Pierre Robin was a pioneer in the development such gadgets. Professor Balters followed up his studies and introduced the Bionator, which is still used nowadays virtually in it's original form.

A further development – by Dr. von Treuenfels – is the bionator which is designed specifically for adults. Bionators are on one hand a device for relaxation; and on the other they can be used for breathing problems whilst sleeping (snoring, apnoea, respiratory gaps). They can also be useful for patients with head joint problems.

The bionator is designed to keep the lower jaw in a forward position; this prevents the soft tissue in the pharyngeal area from collapsing and therefore prevents snoring.

Through the gentle movement and functionality of the bionator, the mouth area is constantly stimulated by a light oscillation which acts as a positive component to the tissue of the teeth, the bones and the soft tissue. This assists the drainage of the lymphatic fluids, relaxes the muscle structure, facilitates the closure of the mouth and therefore restores the full function of the mouth, including the vacuum created within the inner mouth area, which is of great importance when swallowing and head posture.

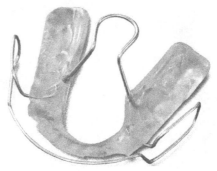

Fig. 35: The Bionator can eliminate the use of harmful external influences which affect the growth of the masticatory organ.

The bionator is used in holistic orthodontics and is a very good device to combat the possible harm caused by breathing through the mouth. It is an element in functional orthodontics which eliminates the use of intrusive harmful components which may obstruct or damage the growth of the jaw.

3.4.3.3   Function Regulator According To Fränkel

A function regulator according to Professor Fränkel is a functional orthodontic device which at an early stage of treatment can have a positive influence on the masticatory apparatus.

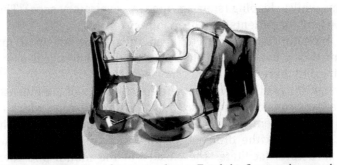

Fig. 36: The functional regulator according to Fränkel influences the growth of the bone of the masticatory apparatus in a positive way.

3.4.3.4   Functional orthodontics

Functional orthodontics are measures which help to improve the function of the mouth. Especially the developement of the jaw is in the focus. Functional orthodontics is best at a young age. Later it is not longer possible to develop the jaw passively with a favourable outcome and active measurements need to be taken.

3.4.3.5   Multiband treatment

The multiband treatment is the so called fixed brace. Brackets are being glued onto the teeth, band are fixed onto the side and flexible nickel titanium arches for guiding the brackets and the teeth are being attached. The multiband treatment is a method which guides the teeth and puts them into the right position. Many holistic therapists reject the multiband treatment completely. However, this is not compatible with a differentiated knowledge of orthodontics, because loose devices can not treat every orthodontic problem.

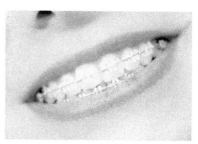

Fig. 37: The multiband treatment ("fixed brace") is also in holistic orthodontics an important treatment measure.

3.4.3.6   Lingualtechnique

The lingualtechnique is an aesthetic refinement of the multiband treatment. Brackets are being fixed onto the inside of the teeth, the wires run also along the inside.

3.4.3.7   Palatal expansion

In some cases, when the teenager is already older and the position of the teeth is very unfavourable, like for example when a cross bite is present, a palatal expansion might be necessary. An expansion plate out of metal is being firmly inserted and via an epansion an enlargement of the upper jaw is being achieved.

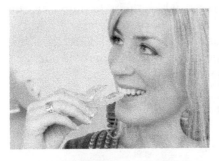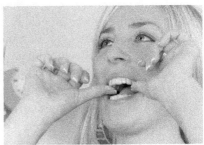

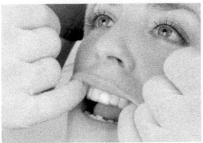

Fig. 38: With thin, invisible splints aesthetically pleasing results can be achieved.

3.4.3.8   Mini-implants

With small implants in orthodontics a good fixation for braces can be achieved. Small implants are for this purpose inserted into the bone and the brace is fixed onto them. After the treatment the mini-implants are being removed.

3.4.3.9   Dental splint orthodontics

With teeth positions which affect the aesthetics it often useful, to treat them with thin splints, which shift the teeth. With small movements of the teeth a great effect can be achieved. We use a system with see through, thin and almost invisible splints.

3.4.4 When should orthodontics be done?

The earlier orthodontics is started, the better. It is easier to achieve changes in the jaw with loose appliances in children. Therefore it is important, to bring children already at the age of 5 to 6 to an orthodontist.

3.5 Dental fracture, dental abrasion, maldevelopment of teeth

Not only caries or periodontities can cause problems in the mouth. A dental fracture is the breakage of a tooth or part of a tooth. This can be caused by an accident, by teeth which have become brittle after root treatment, a false bite, or due to crunching and pressing of the teeth and stones in the food.

If a tooth is broken or a bit of it is broken off, the dentist has to establish whether it is worth saving the tooth and if this is the case, the best treatment has to be established. In the best of cases a plastic filling will do. If the breakage is very big, it might be necessary that the tooth needs a crown. Sometimes a broken tooth needs to be root treated, because the nerve has been damaged.

Unfortunately in some cases a tooth can not be saved and has to be removed.

Dental abrasion is caused by crunching and pressing. This two actions cause the dental enamel and eventually the dentin to be rubbed away. To rub the hard dental enamel and eventually the dentin off, great force is needed. Usually the crunching happens during the night, but it might also occur during the day.

Due to an abrasion of the teeth by crunching and pressing, the teeth and the bone in which the teeth are embedded gets destroyed. Tooth ache, muscle ache, jaw ache, a change of the height of the bite, aesthetic faults and chew and bite problems are the result.

The reasons are usually a wrong bite or orthopedic problems, which rise through the body. This is often in addition to stress and metabolic problems. Even neurological problems can lead to crunching or pressing. Seldom, psychological or neurological reasons are the only cause for dental abrasion.

Dental deformities or misalignements can be inheritry, They also can be caused by an accident, by medicaments, during pregnancy or faulty developements during childhood. Even genetic defects can cause dental deformities or misalignements.

Sometimes small measures are enough to compensate dental deformities or misalignements. If the problems are bigger, like for instance if the teeth are severly deformed or missing, orthodontic and prostetic measures have to be taken.

3.6   TMD – Temporomandibular joint dysfunction and CMD – Craniomandibular dysfunction

3.6.1   What is TMD? And what is CMD?

Temporomandibular joint dysfunction – shortened to – TMD. A complicated name for a complicated matter. "Wikipedia" describes it in short:

"Temporomandibular joint dysfunction (TMD, TMJD) is an umbrella term covering pain and dysfunction of the muscles of mastication (the muscles that move the jaw) and the temporomandibular joints (the joints which connect the mandible to the skull). The most important feature is pain, followed by restricted mandibular movement, and noises from the temporomandibular joints (TMJ) during jaw movement. Although TMD is not life-threatening, it can be detrimental to quality of life, because the symptoms can become chronic and difficult to manage.

TMD is a symptom complex rather than a single condition, and it is thought to be caused by multiple factors. However, these factors are poorly understood, and there is disagreement as to their relative importance. There are many treatments available, although there is a general lack of evidence for any treatment in TMD, and no widely accepted treatment protocol. Common treatments include provision of occlusal splints, psychosocial interventions like cognitive behavioral therapy, and pain medication or others. Most sources agree that no irreversible treatment should be carried out for TMD.

About 20% to 30% of the adult population are affected to some degree. Usually people affected by TMD are between 20 and 40 years of age, and it is more common in females than males. TMD is the second most frequent cause of orofacial pain after dental pain (i.e. toothache)."

TMD is also called CMD – craniomandibular dysfunction. For a more fundamental understanding we take a look at the term itself:

Cranium means skull in latin,

Mandibula means the lower jaw, and

dysfunction signifies, that the skull and the lower jaw, which are connected via the teeth, the jaw joints and the muscles of the masticatory apparatus, do not properly fit together and therefore cannot function efficiently.

Cranium and Mandibula have their points of attachement in the jaw joints and on the teeth, as seen in the second part "All it needs for it: The craniomandibular joint". Furthermore they are connected via muscles, tendons and ligaments.

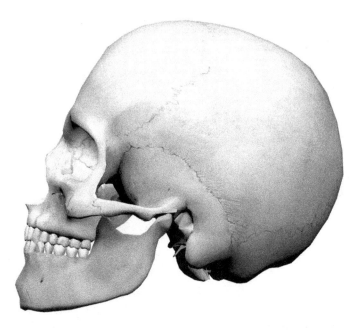

Fig. 39: CMD means the lower jaw does not fit to the skull, the bite is wrong, the jaw joints are misplaced and the muscles of the masticatory apparatus are tense.

3.6.2 Mandibular joint and teeth

The mandibula, the lower jaw is a bone by itself with two joint heads, (like already described in chapter 2), it is connected with the skull base via the jaw joints, but it does not belong to the skull.

The joint heads of the lower jaw come as a pair, which is very special to them. They are siamese twins – the form a stereojoint. Whenever one of them is doing something, the other one is also doing something. This means, that if there is a problem on one side, the other side too does not function properly.

Those two joint heads meet in the sockets, which are placed directly in the base of the skull, in the temporal bone.

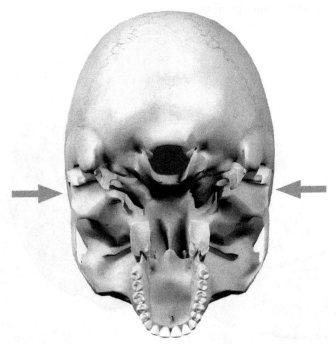

Fig. 40: The sockets of both jaw joints are placed within the base of the skull.

Health is only possible with a balanced bite and jaw joint. This theory is cemented by new studies and case examples. Like e. g. the manager, who, after a burn out syndrome, when all the other therapies did not show any effect, was helped with a bite splint therapy. As well as the young working mother which could follow her daily tasks again after a bite improvement.

Especially important is the craniomandibular dysfunction therapy for patients which got injured in accidents, e. g. the head joints or the cervical spine in whiplash traumas.

By taking the bite pressure from the jaw joints, less force is being diverted onto the head joints and the cervical vertebrae joints, and therefore they are being relieved.

The craniomandibular dysfunction (CMD) is a wide spread illness in our population. We analyze the fault within the bite and its repercussions on the body. We treat the false bite with bite splints, orthodontics and dentures. The symptoms are being treated with CMD-pain therapy. The correction of the bite goes hand in hand with the corrections of the posture.

Illnesses of the jaw are not rare. Even children suffer from CMD. We distinguish between degenerative problems within the jaw joint, malpositions in the jaw joint, immunological problems within the jaw joint and injuries. The degenerative problems occur usually due to strains in the jaw joint. These strains can be due to a wrong bite, severe muscle tensions and posture problems (e.g. problems with the cervical spine). This can causes on the long run "wear and tear". The bone structures, like mandibular joint head or socket, can deteriorate, the ligaments in the jaw joints can wear out and the joint disc the "discus articularis" can show signs of wear and tear or can suffer perforation.

A forward displacement of the joint disc can also occur. A restriction in the joint and in its function would be the result. Misalignments in the jaw joint can be caused by muscular problems and posture problems.

Autoimmune diseases or hormonal problems can also lead to jaw joint problems or illnesses.

Blows to the jaw, injuries caused by accidents like a whiplash, and other accidents can cause permanent damage to the jawjoint.

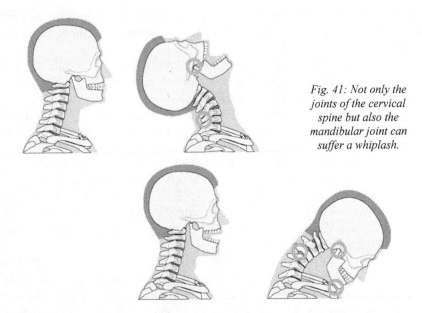

Fig. 41: Not only the joints of the cervical spine but also the mandibular joint can suffer a whiplash.

The positions of the teeth are responsible for the position of the mandibular joint. If for instance a backbite is present, together with e. g. a deep bite to the left, we got a compression on both sides, which is worse on one side.

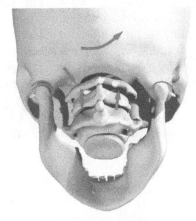

Fig. 42: With an uneven bite the strain on the jaw joints is uneven.

Almost everybody suffers from some problem with misaligned teeth or the other (even after an orthodontic treatment), therefore everybody can potentially suffer from CMD.

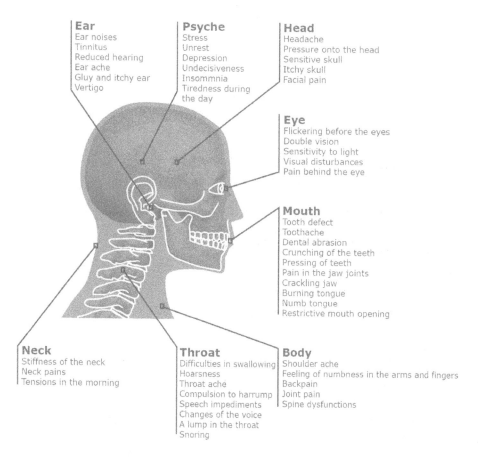

Ear
Ear noises
Tinnitus
Reduced hearing
Ear ache
Gluy and itchy ear
Vertigo

Psyche
Stress
Unrest
Depression
Undecisiveness
Insommnia
Tiredness during the day

Head
Headache
Pressure onto the head
Sensitive skull
Itchy skull
Facial pain

Eye
Flickering before the eyes
Double vision
Sensitivity to light
Visual disturbances
Pain behind the eye

Mouth
Tooth defect
Toothache
Dental abrasion
Crunching of the teeth
Pressing of teeth
Pain in the jaw joints
Crackling jaw
Burning tongue
Numb tongue
Restrictive mouth opening

Neck
Stiffness of the neck
Neck pains
Tensions in the morning

Throat
Difficulties in swallowing
Hoarsness
Throat ache
Compulsion to harrump
Speech impediments
Changes of the voice
A lump in the throat
Snoring

Body
Shoulder ache
Feeling of numbness in the arms and fingers
Backpain
Joint pain
Spine dysfunctions

Fig. 43: CMD can cause many different symptoms.

3.6.3 Head- and bodyposition

Cranium and Mandibula can also be affected by other influences. A muscular dysfunction can be a crucial factor in developing CMD.

From all muscles, the masticatory muscles and the muscles of the neck have the greatest interconnection with the brain. They have to make sure, that the head is in an upright position. Especially in children, where the relation between head and body is greater, it is a big factor in the development of problems and malfunctions.

In the USA, CMD is called TMD. Temporo-Mandibular-Disorders. There, another illness is differenciated, MPD. It stands for "Myofascial Pain Dysfunction Syndrome".

"Myofascial Pain Dysfunction Syndrome" is the illness of the masticatory muscles and its consequences. I include TMD and MPD in the spectrum of CMD.

The position of the teeth and the jaw are connected to the head position. The position of the teeth and the jaw joints are, amongst other things, responsible for the position of the head joints and the vertebra of the column.

3.6.4 What is the perfect body posture?

According to Prof. Wilhelm Balters, the inventor of the orthodontic appliance "Bionator", there is a line running through the foramen magnum of the skull (that is the hole in the skull through which the spinal marrow extravasates from the brain), through the 1st and 2nd cervical vertebra (head joint), the 12th thoracic vertebra, the hip joint and the foot joint.

There is a beautiful methapher in yoga, an angel which, with a thread in the head, pulls the whole body in an upright position. The "angel thread" is like the "threat from above", from the Alexander technique. Both techniques are aimed, like the Balters line, to pull the body up, to achieve and upright and straight posture. The exercises, that follow these techniques, can be done alone. This leads to an improvement of the posture, mainly in the head and neck area.

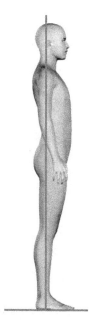

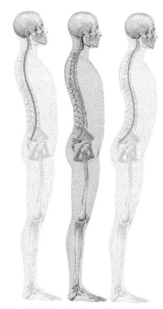

*Fig. 44: Perpendicular through the body
axis when the body is in an optimal
position.*

*Fig. 45: The position of the teeth can
severely influence the spine.*

The position of the feet is also to consider. The feet should be firmly on the ground. This means, that all five toes, the balls, the heals and the outsides of the feet, every part of the feet, should have contact with the floor whilst standing up. When walking, all these parts should be used. Only the foot arch does not touch the ground. The stomach should be tense and the pelvis should be tilted backwards through tensioning of the bottom muscles.

When CMD is diagnosed, the whole posture should be looked at. It is important to distinguish between ascending and descending causes.

Descending causes means that the bite influences the posture. Ca. 80% of all causes are descending, this might be due to the extremely high nerve density in the craniomandibular system. Ascending causes means that the posture is worsened by causes which are further down the body, like for example foot problems, and this again has an impact on the jaw and the bite. The ascending causes account for ca. 20% of the problems.

Usually there is a mixed situation. Due to the nerve density in the masticatory apparatus and the effect of the bite, I consider the treatment of the bite paramount. The bite should first be adjusted with a splint, before posture problems should be dealt with. This enables a more precise treatment. The splint needs to be in accordance to the successes in the treatment of the body.

The following connections between bite and posture can be drawn:

1. Back bite and deep bite cause often a head forward position with a hyperlordosis of the spinal column (forward inclination). If there is a compression onto the jaw joints, like it is the case for the backbite, a forward twisting of the skull may be the result. A backward shift of the joint surface underneath the skull might be the consequence. This might result in a hyperlordosis with a forward position of the head.

2. An uneven bite, which is deeper on one side, can additionally cause a head inclination to the other side.

3. An open bite is often combined with a compression within the head joint, which then results in the spur (Dens axis) of the second cervical vertebrae pushing too far into the brainstem.

4. A forebite can cause a head backwards posture with the cervical spine being too straight. This might result in a pulling force in the jaw joints, a twist of the skull and a forward shift of the joint surface. Because the first two top cervical vertebra (C1 and C2) are tightly connected via ligaments, such twisst are pulling the whole cervical spine. A wrong bite can therefore lead to a malposition of the cervical spine.

5. A one-sided crossbite can cause the head to tilt to the other side.

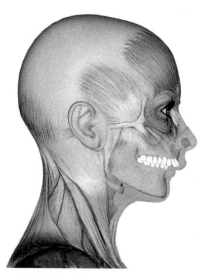

Fig. 46: A backbite favours a forward head position.

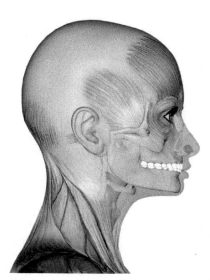

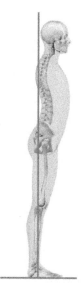

Fig. 47: A deep bite results also in a forward head position. If the bite is asymmetrical and deeper on one side, a malposition of the head to one side might be the result. See Fig. 49, a crossbite can result in a similar malposition of the head.

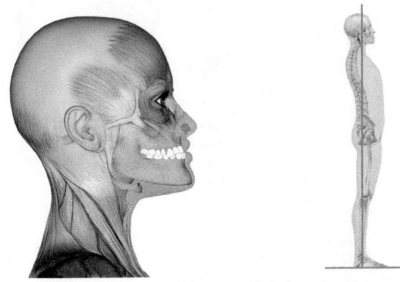

Fig. 48: A forebite favours a head position too far back over the spine.

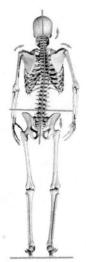

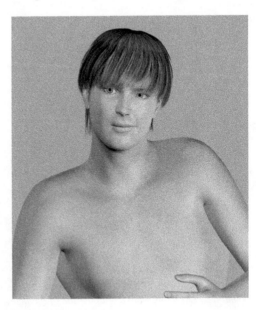

Fig. 49: A crossbite favours a sideward malposition.

When looking at missaligned teeth, missalignedments of the head joints should also be looked at. They are often affected by problems of the bite. It has to be taken into account how the skull is positioned on the head joints. There might be a too forward or too backward twist.

There can be a sideways displacement of the skull in relation to the head joints. There might also be a compression, or a downwards or upwards pull on just one side or both sides. If these problems of the head joints do not improve with splint therapy, the causes must be somewhere else in the body. For this reason, it might be a good idea, to start parallel to the first bite splint therapeutic measures like osteopathy or a manual therapy.

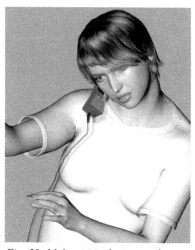

Fig. 50: Malposition during work can cause severe posture problems.

An improvement of the posture is also important. Only this one will ensure the optimum bite for the patient.

In order to improve one's posture, it is important to stop bad habits. If, for example, someone always buts the telephone receiver between the ear and the shoulder, this can result in permanent posture problems.

Especially bad is a bad posture in front of the computer. Especially the asymmetry caused by using a mouse can cause severe posture problems.

Very bad for the posture is flat breathing through the mouth. Hereby, the cervical spine is not stretched far enough backwards, the thorax and the lungs cannot properly expand and breathing is not as efficient as it could be, because the breathing is not done to the full. Because it is connected via the ribs, this affects the whole spine. The thorax is not stretched enough, and the muscles between the rips shrink and become tense. Other muscles are then used as a support, like e. g. the muscles used for turning the neck or the neck muscles themselves. This leads to tensions in the throat and neck muscles. Far reaching posture problems and severe muscle tensions are the consequence.

Mouth breathing with the tongue positioned wrongly, is one of the main reasons for tooth displacements.

A particularity of the cervical vertebra C1 and C2, is the absence of intervertebral discs. One can assume, that the intervertebral discs of the head joints C1 and C2 can be found in the craniomandibular system, in the bite and the jaw joints. The reason for this is described above, they adapt to every situation.

The head weighs roughly as much as a bowling ball. If the head is held in a forward position, one can imagine, that an imbalance develops. If you got problems with the neck or the spine, you'll probably have a problem with the bite the jaw joints and/or the head posture.

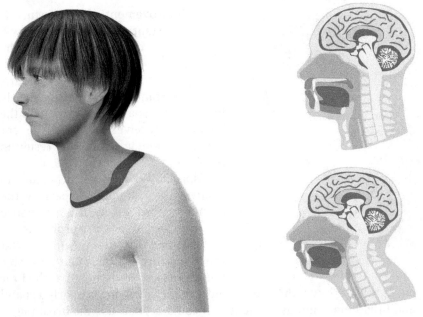

Fig. 51: The biomechanics of the head posture is very complex. The heavy head is being balanced on top of the fragile spine, with the sensory organs, the nerves and the muscles. If only one component of this complex system is out of balance, the whole system is affected. The distance between atlas and axis in the invertebrate extensions, shows the extent of the head twist, this can be seen via x-rays. If the angle between the two invertebrate extensions is normal, the head rest in an upright position on top of the spine. If the angle is narrowed, a forward twist of the skull is the result; if the angle is widened, a backwards twist of the skull is the result. The mandibular joints are also connected to spine via the Ganglion of the trigeminus nerve.

3.6.5 Symptoms of CMD

CMD is not an illness, but a dysfunction. It can cause many symptoms, and can develop into an illness. CMD can be very treacherous, because many symptoms don't seem to have anything to do with the teeth, the bite, the jaw joint or the masticatory muscles.

If one looks at the most common symptoms of CMD, it is self explanatory as to why CMD is overseen so often:

Symptoms shown in the teeth:
Pressing of the teeth, grinding of the teeth, defects of the dental necks, tooth ache, sensitive tooth necks, retrieving gums, wrong bite, numbness (teeth, lips, tongue, cheek), burning on the mouth mucus, problems with chewing, tooth movements, loosening of teeth, grinding down of a tooth, lips can not be closed due to one tooth.

Mandibular joint symptoms:
Pains in the mandibular joints, cracking of the jaw joint, grinding sounds in the jaw joint, the mouth cannot be opened, pains in the mandibular joint, tensions when waking up in the morning.

Pains:
Head ache, neck ache, facial pain, head pressure, stiffness of the neck, stiffness of other muscles, sensitive skull, itchy skull, back pain.

Symptoms of the eyes:
Visual disturbances, flickering before the eyes, painful eyes, sensitivity to light.

Ear symptoms:
Tinitus (sounds in the ear), deafness, ear pains, feeling of a "blogged up" ear, itchy ear, dizziness.

Throat symptoms:
Problems in swallowing, croakiness, throat ache, compulsion to burp, voice problems, speech problems, a "lump" in the throat.

Breathing:
Mouth breathing, snoring, tight thorax.

Symptoms shoulders, arms, back:
Numb arms, numb hands, shoulder pains, back pains, fibromyalgia (fibre-muscle pain), joint pains.

Psychological symptoms:
Work related stress, family related stress, restlessness, grumpiness, mood swings, depression, indecision, insomnia.

3.6.6 How does CMD develop

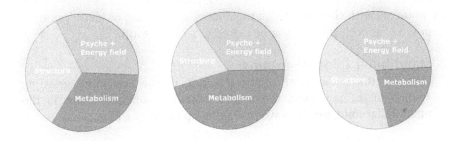

Fig. 52: A healthy person holds a balance. If in one area the balance is tipped, an illness can develop.

CMD has always multiple causes. That means that CMD is only then symptomatic when different factors come together. Sometimes, CMD can be caused by only one factor, which is very severe. Normally a patient with CMD has various things which contribute to developing CMD.

It is important, when treating CMD, not only to solve the problems of the bite, but to find all the other triggering factors. Treatment will be done by the dentist or somebody else how is trained to deal with the specific problematic. This is called interdisciplinary working within the medical network. That means, if a patient has not only tooth and jaw problems, but also a posture problem, it makes sense to include an orthopaedic doctor and also a physiotherapist in the treatment of the patient. If there is a psychological problematic, a psychotherapist is to consult, which then can treat the patient.

A stroke does not suddenly happen overnight, and also CMD does not develop overnight. It is a chronic degenerative illness, it can take years for CMD to cause visible problems. Because CMD is not a simple infect, we have to find the various causes.

The jaw is within a person and therefore this person has to be taken into consideration. I am going to divide them in four aspects:

The structure of a person,
his/her metabolism,
his/her psyche and
his/her energy field.

Depending on how severe a malfunction is, the effect are more or less severe. Rarely all malfunctions are equally severe. It is very important, to investigate everything properly in order to be able to find the right therapy and the right interdisciplinary collaboration.

One can compare the development of CMD with an overfull barrel or an overflowing dam. The body can compensate for al long time. If eventually too many factors converge, the barrel overflows or, even worse, the dam breaks.

That means one day you'll wake up with an unbearable headache and you wonder why it persists. Maybe you already had a lot of problems beforehand, which

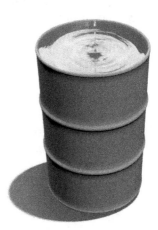

Fig. 53: If many factors converge, the "barrel" is overflowing, and CMD develops.

your body was able to compensate, but suddenly your body is unable to, and severe problems are the result.

3.6.6.1 The structure of a person or functional disturbances

With CMD, there is always an underlying structural problem. Like mentioned above, structural problems are: a wrong bite, malocclusion or malposition of the jaw.

Malposition of the jaw means that the teeth of the upper jaw do not line up correctly with the lower jaw (occlusion). The occlusion can be compared to a table. It has to be on four legs to be stable. The teeth have to fit together properly in order to have the muscles and joints in the right position. This enables for instance proper chewing and swallowing.

Malposition of the jaw means, that the mandibular joints are in the wrong position, the movement of the jaws is faulty, the skull is in the wrong position. All this results in health problems. The teeth determine the position of the jaw joints.

When a malocclusion is present, the muscles are in the wrong position and tensions are the consequence.

Every body part has a corresponding area in the brain. The area in the brain which is responsible for the craniomandibular system is, in relation, the biggest of all of them. This explains the severely negative effects a malocclusion has for neurological diseases.

The loss of a tooth can imbalance the whole neuromuscular system. Due to the gap the stimuli to the nerves and the muscles and therefore to the brain are different. If, after a while, other teeth move into the gap, the situation can worsen even further.

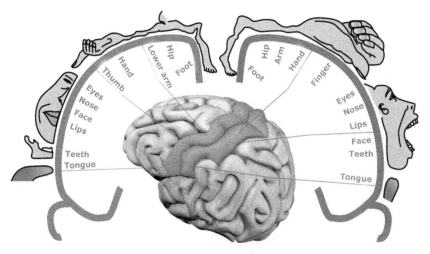

HOMUNCULUS
Sensomotoric Area

Fig. 54: The area of the brain which is responsible for the masticator apparatus is extremely big compared to other body parts.

A faulty denture or faulty orthodontics can be the reason for a malocclusion. Misaligned teeth can be the cause, but also wrongly designed dentures can cause the tongue not to function properly, this can have devastating effects.

One swallows ca. 2000 times a day, and every time the lower jaw is pressed onto the upper jaw. If the bite is faulty it affects the muscles, the head posture and the whole body structure with all its nerves. This is called functional disturbance. It can be compared to a Ganglion. If one wears non fitting shoes for years, the anatomy of the bones and muscles of the feet change.

The head is extremely heavy. It weighs between 7 and 13 kg and is balanced on the delicate spine. To guarantee for a balanced hold and to be able to execute difficult head movements, it needs jaw muscles as well as the anterior and rear neck muscles, which are also known as accessory chewing muscles.

That means that the so called masticatory apparatus is also the apparatus to hold the head and which controls all head movements.

If one imagines shortened or stretched muscles caused by malocclusion, one can imagine that it results in posture problems and related illnesses like slipped discs, nerve illnesses, dizziness etc. Severe muscle tensions can also be a result, these can cause via so called trigger points severe pains.

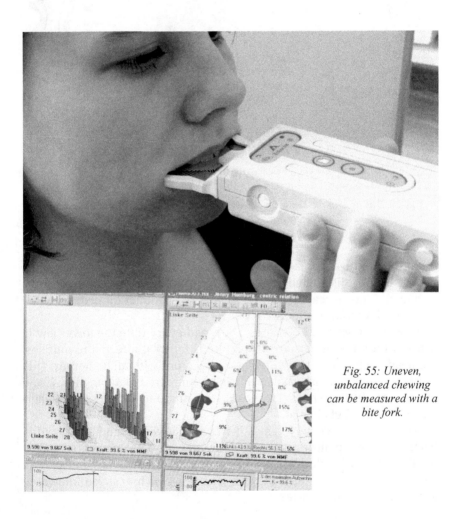

Fig. 55: Uneven, unbalanced chewing can be measured with a bite fork.

Trigger points are muscle tensions and hardenings the size of lentils. They trigger tensions to the whole muscle and are often responsible for pain.

Trigger points are not in the area where the pain is felt. They produce a radiating pain. It might even be the case that trigger points produce pains in the area of the teeth. Often such pain ends in a complete mistreatment, a root treatment of the tooth.

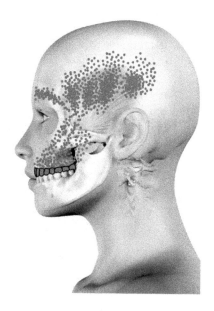

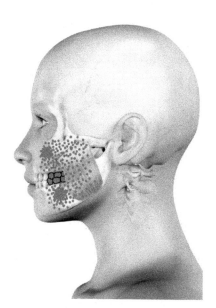

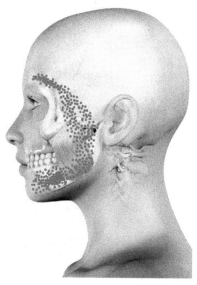

Fig. 56: Trigger points in the masticatory muscles cause pain in a different location.

85

It can be concluded, that a malocclusion has two consequences:

1. It changes the position of the jaw joints and causes therefore an extreme pressure to the very sensible surroundings.

2. It twists or bends the jaw in a position where it is permanently tense. This can affect the muscles of the face, the head, the neck, the back and of the shoulders. This can cause pain. Due to these tensions, a deteriorating bite can be the result.

This is the reason as to why a correct bite is very important. Subsequently I will explain, what such a difficult situation, with muscles out of control, has to do with problems with the metabolism, the psyche and the energetic field.

3.6.6.2 What has a craniomandibular dysfunction to do with the metabolism?

Craniomandibular dysfunctions and its symptoms can be amplified by metabolic problems. A craniomandibular dysfunction can be symptom free for years. Due to certain metabolic factors a decompensatory situation can occur after years of compensation. The following factors seems to be responsible:

- Wrong foods
- Regular use of medication
- Inherited or acquired metabolic problems
- Deterioration of the metabolism due to age (e. g. menopause)
- Poisoning
- Over-acidification of the tissue
- Intollerances, allergies
- False breathing
- Permanent stress (often caused by CMD, can be responsible for changes in the metabolism)

I would like to especially point out the hormonal relations with the craniomandibular system. A malocclusion can influence the hormonal metabolism. The bite directly affects the frontal muscles of the neck, this might cause too much pressure on the sensitive thyroid and this might affect its functionality.

Wrong pressure in the skull and breathing through the mouth as well as too little air through the nose and the pharyngeal tonsils can cause problems in the pituitary gland, which is responsible for the hormonal system in the body.

Problems within the nervous system due to a false bite can cause a false release of stress hormones. A problem of the autonomous nervous system due to mechanical interference might also occur. This can cause or favour reactions like e.g. cardiac arrhythmias or digestive problems.

A further point is the breathing. Breathing is essential for living and should be at its optimum to guarantee a healthy metabolism. Some malocclusion can severely affect the breathing and lead to considerable problems.

The connection between the masticatory muscles and the jaw joint with the receptors of the sex hormones oestrogen and progesterone is also very interesting.

In the masticatory muscles and also in the mandibular joint are many recipients for sex hormones. If, during menopause they decrease, difficulties with the masticatory muscles and the mandibular joint can be the result. It can also affect men, but this is rarely the case because testosterone seems to have a protective influence.

3.6.6.3 To fight through life, to remain persistent and other psychological factors which might be related to CMD

CMD was associated for a long time to the area of psychosomatic (soma = body). It signifies that illnesses, which have a psychological origin, spread to the body. Examples of illnesses with psychosomatic origins are gastric ulcers and high blood pressure. It is an important to know, that if there is a problem of the psyche, (stress, tension), bad illnesses can be the result.

We know today that CMD has usually a structural origin and that psychological problems develop out of CMD problems. It starts with a malocclusion and/or a malposition of the mandibular joint, this causes stress, which then develops into a psychological problem. This can only be solved by solving the structural problem. If the psychological factor is very severe is should also be treated.

Often patients develop bad habits due to CMD. For instance a wrong posture to avoid pain, crunching, pressing, wrong muscle tensions or other bad habits with the mouth. These should be resolved with behavioural therapeutic measures.

Head and facial pains affect us more than pains in other areas. The reason for this is, that the brain and its life support structures are very close to the mouth. This scares patients more than just a toe which hurts. This fear is often intensified by the fear of the unknown. The patient does not know what's wrong with him/her and that is very scary.

This is the reason as to why MPD (Myofascial Pain Dysfunction Syndrome) is considered the second illness, the illness behind CMD.

CMD-patients are often under great stress. Stress is being judged by how a patient reacts to Stressors. This means, that there are great differences in how patients respond to stress situations. These differences depend on various factors, like sex, age, nourishment, fitness, personality and habits.

An emotional problematic opens up a vicious cycle. Triggered by a structural problem which then leads to emotional stress. This stress enhances the structural problem with pressing, grinding, wrong posture or muscle tension and enhances again the emotional factor.

3.6.6.4 The energy field of a person – not only biochemistry works but also physics

a. The pollution with electricity at work, a place for relaxation, or in bed is indisputably important. It is a known factor, that even if appliances are turned off, an electromagnetic field persists, which can interfere with the physical interaction of the body with its cells. This can result in health problems, mainly in the neurological area. I advice my patients to take a closer look at their living and working environment and, if necessary, to have them investigated by a geobiological adviser or an experienced electrician. The bed should always be free of electromagnetic fields. This won't usually be completely possible with regards to the working space, but a lot can be achieved by some shielding off.

b. More controversial is the pollution through earth radiation. Before the Second World War a lot of research has been done about it. One believes, that as a result of distortions in the earth, water veins and other structures, physical forces occur, which can influence the body and its functions. If somebody is interested in further reading, I will point out further literature. An interesting fact is, that already Sauerbruch told his tumour patients to change the position of their beds.

c. Scars are also an energetic burden. If one is to assume that there are not only biochemical forces, but also physical ones and if one considers, that healthy tissue flows are important for the bodily functions, one can imagine the impact of scars. Often there is a simple scar, that can interfere with the biodynamic processes of the muscles and the surrounding structures. In Chinese and Indian medicine so called meridians are important in keeping healty. These meridians are thought to be physical tissue flows.

Scars can be serious blocages in the body. A scar is formed by the destruction of the collagenous tissue net of the skin, it is then replaced by tissue of lesser quality. As cause of the injury nerves are disconnected and energy flows interrupted. Painful scars have too much energy, scars which cause no pain have too little energy. The latter can be improved by toning, e. g. via EVA. Painful scars need to be relieved of energy for instance via acupuncture. Furthermore, scars can successfully treated by bioresonance, magnetic field therapy and with creams. Especially when CMD is diagnosed, it is important to get rid of all negative influences caused due to scars.

Functional disturbances are not considered enough. Even though it seems to be a very obvious thing. If something in the body is not straight, the result is stress in this area. If one body part is not straight, usually everything is distorted. And if nothing is straight, all is more or lessvunder stress you must have experienced trolleys with a lopsided wheel. You will not manage to make the other wheels go straight. Or, if we compare the body with a house, where a supporting wall has been taken away, it will collapse! These examples might be descriptive, but can't describe the full extent of the impact, because a shopping trolley and a house do not have the complexity of a human organism.

Furthermore, a house is a static object, humans are as well as static also dynamic.

These two metaphors can depict, what I want to explain. It want to show you that a functional problem in the jaw area, like for instance a wrongly proportioned jaw, can have drastic consequences for the whole body. This false proportion is called craniomandibular dysfunction. Short CMD.

The body can compensate for this disequilibrium for a long time. This favours an asymmetry even further. Often, after due time, a decomposition of the problematic situation and symptoms of illness manifest itself.

Functional problems in the jaw area can trigger or favour many illnesses. Orthopaedic, neurological, otorhinolaryngologycal, sleeping disorder related, craniological, internist, endocrinological and other problems have often a craniomandibular dysfunction as a main trigger or as additional trigger.

More than 50 % of all visits to doctors are due to head-, neck-, shoulder or back pain. If you are one of these patients and you did not find any help or only little help, this book could be interesting for you. Alone in Germany more than 30% of all inhabitants suffer form chronical headaches and many of them could be helped with a CMD treatment.

Usually one goes to a doctor, but if he/she does not get rid of these problems, a visit to the dentist might be advisory. Knowing of the connection of CMD and its treatments. If you heard sentences like "it is psychological", or "it is age related", than you should not leave it there. You should rather think if it could be a dysfunction in the jaw area and you should get it treated by a dentist.

Pain and chronic diseases can and should be treated and there is often a chance to achieve this, when different suitable therapies are undertaken and the functional disturbance is taken into consideration.

3.6.7 What to do if I got CMD?

3.6.7.1 Functional Analysis

Often is the bite responsible for many problems throughout the whole body. To establish exactly where the problem within the bite lies and what the repercussions are, a good analysis is necessary.

It can be distinguished between an analysis with regards to only dentistry and an analysis considering the whole body relating to the bite.

From a dental point of view, the dentist examines the masticatory muscles, the position as well as the movements of the mandibular joint, the malposition of the bite and the bite defects.

If the bite is examined holistically, one can also include the posture, the spine, the muscle force, the vegetative strain, relations with sleep and strains on the food. There is a discussion going on, that changes in the bite can have a big impact on the whole body.

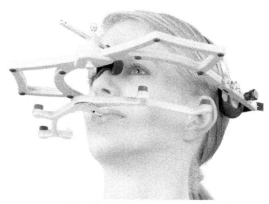

Fig. 57: Before treating CMD a dental functional analysis is necessary.

3.6.7.2 Bite splint

If there is a wrong bite, so called bite splints have to be used. They cause a relaxation of the muscles and the mandibular joint. Different types of bite splints are distinguished.

3.6.7.2.1 Neuromuscular myocentric bite splints

A lopsided, wrongly positioned, or asymmetrical bite affects the muscles in their proper position. If one wants to treat the symptoms of a wrong bite from the start, the muscles need to be relaxed.

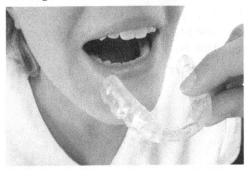

Fig. 58: During night time, a bite splint with a relaxing effects, is the best option.

This can only be achieved with bite splints, which ensure a more symmetrical and even bite. A relaxation in the sense of a stretching of the tense and compressed muscles makes sense. It can be achieved via different relaxation methods like transcutaneous nerve stimulation (TENS), osteopathy, and similar methods. The muscles are controlled and measured with surface electromyography.

3.6.7.2.2 Bite Rising Splints

Before a bite is corrected with prosthetic measures or with orthodontics, it needs to be relaxed and evened out with bite splints. Prior, they should be individually measured.

We use electromyography and cinematography (exact measuring of the masticatory muscles with regards to the symmetry and equal force on both sides, as well as measuring the movement of the jaws). Only after a certain settling time and successively an adaption time, can the new bite, definitely changed with dentures or changes in the chewing surface.

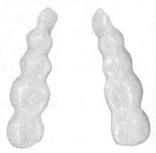

Fig. 59: During daytime the bite is optimized with day splints.

3.6.8 CMD-pain therapy

CMD is often responsible for chronic pains which can affect the whole body. The therapy with bite splints and interdisciplinary additional therapie, like for instance osteopathy has to be checked regularly. The initial complaints are being carefully checked via questionnaires and, based on the new situation. Finally, the new situation is explained to each patient individually. The instruction encompasses further therapies and other advices like tips on the correct nourishment or exercises.

3.6.9 Posture and CMD

The bite and the position of the teeth have got a lot to do with the posture. Problems within the craniomandibular system might have something to do with a wrong body posture. Therefore, analyzing the posture is of great importance when treating CMD.

Therefore we take pictures of the patient's posture at regular intervals. When comparing the pictures, the success of the treatment can be seen.

An improvement of the posture is achieved by improving the bite with excercises, osteopathy and treatments of the feet.

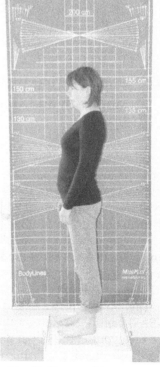

Fig. 60: Picture of the patient's posture.

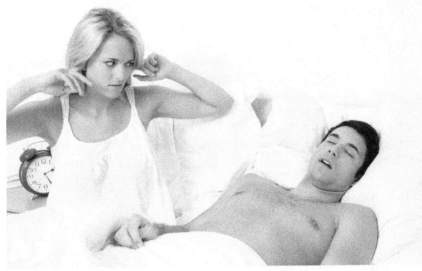

Fig. 61: Snoring is irritating and unhealthy.

3.7 Anti snoring therapy without mask or operation and with additional snoring splints from the dentist.

Snoring is loud and disturbing. This can have far reaching consequences. The partner does not get any sleep and gets ill, the holiday together is no longer possible because one cannot afford two hotel rooms. The person which snores is often embarrassed because it disturbs all the surrounding people, e. g. in mountain huts.

Snoring can also cause illnesses. This occurs when, during sleeping, the air is cut off. This is the so called sleeping apnoea. Sleeping apnoea can cause serious illnesses like a heart attack or other heart- or circulatory illnesses.

The breathing gaps and other sleep related breathing problems (SBAS) can be treated by the dentist with snoring splints. The splints are being put in the upper and lower jaw and stop the soft tissue inside the throat from collapsing. The splint helps to improve snoring and stops the gaps during breathing. No mask and no operation is necessary.

3.7.1 How do I know if my type of snoring is bad for my health?

Appliances which can be borrowed from the praxis and taken home, during the night, these apparatus can then monitor the breathing and also the the cardiovascular system.

With some appliances, sleep phases can be measured exactly. This enables us to see when the patient is in a slow-wave sleep phase. When suffering from sleep apnoea or tooth grinding, the patient sleeps but only lightly. This means they do not enter in a slow-wave sleep phase, and this in the long run affects one's health. The appliance has got a great electrode with three leads. This is being stuck on the patients' forehead and measures how the patient sleeps and if he/she goes through all the sleeping phases. These type of monitoring corresponds to a very simple EEG (electroencephalogram).

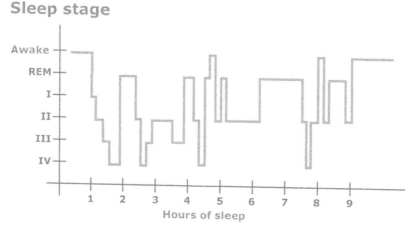

Fig. 62: With a hypnogram the sleep stages can be measured.

After looking at the results in his/her praxis, the dentist can conclude whether a treatment is necessary or not. At the same time he/she can follow the success of the therapy better.

It's equally important to screen sleep related breathing problems which occur during the night. With a further appliance one can diagnose snoring, as well as breathing- heart and circulatory problems. In severe cases the patient should be referred to a sleeping laboratory or a respirologist. There it can be tested, if the treatment with dental appliances is successful and if the respiratory gaps or the cardio-vascular interferences are improving.

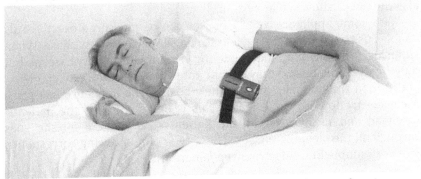

Fig. 63: A screening with Apnealink enables to measure the type of snoring.

The appliances consists of a belt, nose glasses to measure the air which is breathed in, and a fingerclip to measure the heart frequency as well as the oxygen saturation. This is called respiratory dynamic pressure measurement and pulse oximetry.

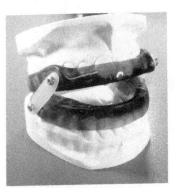

There are different snoring splints. One cannot say that one is best. They need to be individually chosen for each patient.

The production of quality snoring splints is costly, therefore it is possible to check the effectiveness with a test set of snoring splints.

Fig. 64: Upper- and lower jaw are being joined, therefore the lower jaw cannot fall backwards, and this frees the airways.

3.8   Treatment of children

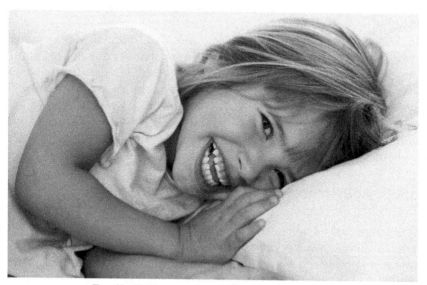

Fig. 65: Children need sensitivity during treatments.

Children are very special patients. They have to be treated with special respect. This involves a lot of time. In my praxis we tray to fulfil the needs of the children and their parents without time pressure and without the use of anaesthetics. Only with consideration for the child and its parents, dentistry for children can successfully be realised.

Children have to understand what is done to them. It is important to explain them everything and to not lie to them. If the trust in the dentist is gone it often remains for the rest of ones live. Surely a playful approach is sometimes advisable, nevertheless, children appreciate if they are taken serious and they have to be kept informed.. It is important to give the child the possibility to take decisions, otherwise helplessness will become a problem during treatment.

If you are sensitive, caring and patient which children, it is normally not necessary to treat them with soforics and silver crowns.

3.9   The icing on the cake –
What is special about holistic dentistry

In holistic dentistry the treatment is not just "normal" like at other dentists. Measures which go beyond dentistry are taken, and most importantly the reasons for the problem are being examined and to avoid having the same problem again in the future. Not only are the symptom being dealt with, but also look the underlying causes for the disease. During treatment, methods are being used which might not withstand scientific criteria, but in the praxis they often lead to a better and quicker healing process. "The success proves one right."

3.9.1 Holistic treatment of teeth and gums

Food plays an important part in the development of tooth and gum related illnesses. Also other medical causes, like hormonal problems, intestinal problems or orthopaedic causes can be the reason for tooth and gum problems. Through the knowledge of holistic dentistry and in collaboration with holistic doctors and therapists, it is possible not only to treat tooth and gum symptoms, but to establish the causes and to deal with them.

Breathing can be responsible for plaque. If breathing occurs only through the mouth, plaque is formed quicker.

A non favourable tooth position can render the cleaning more difficult and also favour the formation of plaque. Certain medicaments can have drastic consequences for the health of the mouth and the dental health. Holistic prophylaxis requires a very thorough initial questioning of the patient. It is not enough to only deal with matters concerning the mouth and the teeth, but it is also necessary to collect all other medical and human factors to get an overall picture of the situation. This is the only way to maintain a holistic overview.

To ensure healthy teeth and healthy gums, it is necessary to have an individual prophylaxis.

3.9.1.1 The Individual Prophylaxis - Individual Risk Assessment

Prevention to maintain healthy teeth encompasses the analysis as to where dental problems could have their origin. Different measures ensure the assessment of the individual risk to suffer from dental illnesses. An individual prophylaxis (IP) is recommended, when assessing the individual risk to suffer from dental illnesses. Individual prophylaxis means that different examinations need to be done to establish the risk of contracting an illness.

The teeth are being checked for plaque and the gums if they are bleeding when lightly touched, this is the documented as plaque- and bleeding rate.

One gropes with a blunt probe at the edge of the gums if there is plaque on the teeth and if the gums are bleeding slightly. Every single tooth is looked at. The resulting index is important for the risk assessment.

If the gums are already diseased and have gingival pockets, the depth of the pockets are being measured and noted down. Afterwards the patient has to produce saliva and this is examined for acids and resistance.

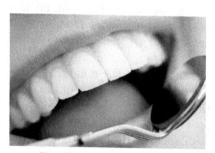

Fig. 66: During an individual prophylaxis, the causes for tooth problems are being looked at.

Saliva plays an important part in the formation of dental illnesses. Saliva can varie from basic to acid, it might deal with acids, which we absorb with our food, better or worse. For instance sour saliva with a weak buffer function, in combination with food rich in carbohydrates can foster caries and peritonitis. Obviously, oral hygiene is herby of great importance. To examine it and as a consequence to instruct a better oral hygiene is an important part of the individual prophylaxis.

If the carious activity is especially high, tests can be done to establish whether there is an increased danger of caries bacteria.

Food advice is again very important. A lot of people do not know what leads to caries and periodontitis. Short chained carbohydrates like e. g. white flour or white sugar are the favoured food of caries and periodontitis bacteria, therefore these and other refined foods foster caries and periodontitis.

Like mentioned above, the connection between breathing problems and dental illnesses is not very known. Permanent breathing through the mouth favours dryness of the teeth and the buccal mucosa. This can lead to caries and periodontitis. Mouth breathing can imbalance the whole acid alkaline balance in the body and consequently lead to an over acidity of the saliva, which then can cause caries and periodontitis. Some patients breath through the nose during the day, but suffer from breathing problems during the night. It might be that patients, which suffer from apnoea, that means respiratory failure during sleep, or allergic patients, breath through their mouth during the night because their nasal mucosa is swollen. They present the same problems like general "mouth – breathers".

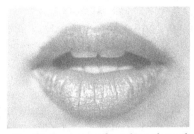

Fig. 67: Permanent breathing through the mouth favours teeth problems.

If the patient is breathing improperly during the night, it can be easily checked out with a mobile appliance, that the patient brings home. If the patient breathes through the mouth even during daytime, this bad habit should be treated with logopedic or speech therapy. If the nose is blocked, a otolaryngologist must additionally be consulted.

3.9.1.2 Professional Odontexesis (PZR) aftercare (Recall)

To create a healthy and clean situation in the mouth and too maintain it, a professional tooth cleaning (PZR) should be done at least twice per year. The PZR does not need to be done by a dentist. It can also be performed by trained dental assistants or dental hygienists.

During PZR the teeth are being thoroughly cleaned with hand tools or ultrasound, they are being polished and remineralised. In holistic dentistry only in exceptional cases single teeth are being fluoridated, because the halogen fluorine can have severe side effects.

The use of fluorid is very controversial. It is proven that it hardens the enamel, but it is critical for the metabolism. Fluorine is in fact a calcium robber. Usually Aminfluorid is being given – which is a very unstable fluorine combination, which will break up immediately once it is in the blood. The free radical fluorine likes to bind calcium, it is a non-reversible bond, with the result that the calcium is no longer available to the body.

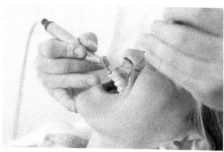

Fig. 68: Two times a year the teeth should be professionally cleaned by a dentist.

For keeping teeth healthy, especially after the treatment of tooth and gum diseases, an appropriate aftercare of the teeth and gums is very important. For this reason a so called recall-system is a necessity. It is established how many times during the treatment the patient has to come back to the praxis for a prophylaxis. If it is time for the agreed appointment, the patient is called or an appointment has been made in advance.

Some patients feel the recall system excertes too much control over them. However, it is proven patients often do not come for prevention to the dental practice, but only when per-problems have already arisen and it is too late for a prevention.

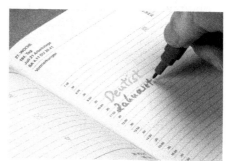

This highlightens the importance of a regular aftercare, controlled and directed by the

Fig. 69: A recall system is very important to keep the teeth healthy.

dental praxis. Especially when existing illnesses of the parodontium are present or if a higher caries risk prevail. It should be individually established how often patients have to come to the praxis to prevent further damage.

If the teeth are discoloured or if their natural tone is of a darker hue, the teeth can be bleached via a professional tooth cleaning. This is done either on the dentist's chair with the direct application of bleaching gel, or with individually fitted rails to use at home. Especially for sensitive teeth bleaching at home is the best way. Bleaching, when it is done correctly and the individual dental and anatomical situation is respected, is unproblematic for the teeth.

Teeth with tight-fitting plaque, that can not be removed by a normal professional tooth cleaning, can be effectively cleaned with dental aesthetic polish. This has to be done by the dentist him/herself, because he/she is working with grinders, special polishing pastes and rapid rotating polishers.

3.9.2 Dental material or medicaments which have not been tested

Dental materials do not come under medicaments but under medical products. That means that they are not subject to the same strict tests as medicaments do. They contain many potentially harmful substances, which can cause health risks to humans. Plastics, catalysts, plasticizers or monomers can be adverse to the immune system of a patient and cause allergies of the type 1 (immediate reaction) and of the type 4 (intolerances). A compatibility test is therefore recommended. The epicutaneous test which is recommended as a guideline can only test for allergies of the type 1. However, if there is an intolerance to dental material only biophysical tests such as kinseology, EAV, etc., or immunological tests such as lymphocyte transformation tests can obtain a result.

3.9.3 Electroacupuncture according to Voll – EAV

Electroacupuncture according to Voll (EAV) is a method to find at an early stage problems within the body via the conductivity of acupuncture points. Furthermore, the EAV helps to find the right medicaments and tooth material. It can be established what the body is missing and what might aggravate it. Suitable homeopathic medicines for treatment can be established via EAV. And also with the weak electric currents from the EAV appliance treatment can be done. EAV is important in finding inflamations within the body. Especially in finding dental focuses.

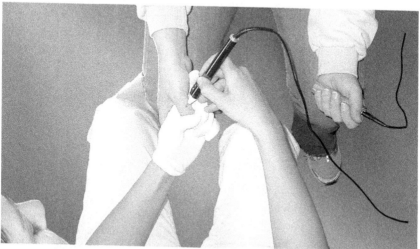

Fig. 70: Electroacupuncture according to Voll (EAV) can test incompatibleness and dental focuses.

3.9.4 A test to detect the transfer of lymphocytes – LTT

LTT is a laboratory method to detect specific reactions of the immune system. It assesses how the immune system reacts to a substance. It is possible to verify immunological and allergological processes within the body, like e. g. drug and dental material incompatibility. Also certain pathogens can be detected.

For the test, blood is taken from the vein. This and the suspected dental material will then be sent to a lab. The reaction of the blood with the tooth material will then be tested. The big advantage for the patient is, that he/she is not sensitized with the tooth material, like it can be the case with the patch test.

3.9.5 Mouth current, or like the mouth became a battery

If, over time, many different metals are placed in the mouth, the saliva reacts as a conductor. Via the saliva, the less precious metal ionises the more precious metal. This leads to a damaging flow of current throughout the mouth. Like it happens in a battery, electric current flows through the mouth, with salvia as a conductor. One can assume, that such electromagnetic fields remain not without effect for nearby anatomical structures, like the brain, the electric flow in the mouth can be measured. If needed, especially older metal is being removed and exchanged by metal free material. This can reduce or eliminate any electric current throughout mouth.

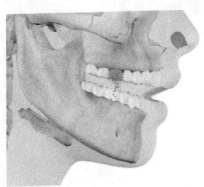

Fig. 71: Due to different metals in the mouth, current flows via the saliva through the mouth.

3.9.6 The reason as to why one can fall ill due to a dental focus

Tooth infections are responsible for chronic diseases throughout the body. For example, a heart, joint, or kidney problems might arise because of a dental focus. Dead teeth whose rootsare either not or only partially filled, are hide holes for bacteria. There, they can multiply undisturbed and then spread via the blood or lymphaticsystem throughout the body. Many teeth die without being noticed by the patient, because they do not hurt. Therefore the patient is not aware of any possible problem, and it could even be, that the patient feels the effects of the dental focus somewhere else in the body.

If the underlying problem is found and consequently treated, often the other disturbances within the body are also cured. This dental treatment is referred to as dental focal reconstruction. From the dental focus tooth bacteria or bacterial toxins might spread throughout the body via the blood stream or the lymphatic system; it might also lead to an energy blockade within the body, This means, that the flow of energy throughout areas of the body might be disturbed by a dead tooth. It is hereby interesting to observe the tooth-organ relationship.

To determine whether a tooth is inflamed, different methods are used in dentistry. First, the appearance of the tooth is examined. If it is black, that might be caused by the death of the nerve, a large filling or a big hole may indicate a dental focus. The dentist taps on the tooth to determine if it is sensitive to touch. This means, that the tooth and the surrounding area is inflamed. An important diagnostic method are X-rays. This helps the dentist to determine if the bone around the tooth tip has been affected. If a tooth does not respond to a tap and if it is not been root treated, this indicates that the tooth is already dead. It is a clear sign for a dead tooth with a dental focus problem. An even more accurate depiction of the tooth can be achieved with a computer tomography.

If conventional methods bring no results, the test methods of biophysical medicine can be used. Here are mainly to mention the above explained electro-acupuncture according to Voll (EAV) and Kinesiology. With these methods possible dental focuses can be found via energetic measurements of the meridians or the muscle chains. One can also establish the exten of the dental focus and its impact on the body, these findings can often be confirmed with conventional methods.

The immunological strain on the body by a dead or endodontically treated tooth can also be tested with the above described lymphocyte transformation test (LTT).

Today, the technique of root treatment is so good, that not every dead tooth needs to be pulled out. The aim should be to perform a very good root treatment of the tooth, as closely to the wall of the root canal as possible. Before this, the canal should be carefully flushed several times to disinfect it. The tooth is then given time to recover and eventually tested if the dental focus is still active.

Dental focus in the upper jaw	1-8	1-7	1-6	1-5-	1-4	1-3	1-2	1-1
Relationship with the immune system	Kidney							
Organs	Heart / Small intestine	Pancreas / Stomach		Lung / Large intestine		Liver/ Bile	Kidney / Bladder	
Cranial cavities	Sine cavern	Maxillary sinus		Ethmoidal air cells		Sphenoidal sinus	Frontal sinus Sphenoidal sinus	
Tonsils	Lingual tonsils	Laryngeal tonsils			Tubal tonsil	Palatine tonsil	Pharyngeal tonsil	
Sensory organs	Inner ear	Tongue Taste			Nose / Smell	Eye (back)	Ear (Chin. 5 Elements)	
Endocrine gland	Anterior pituitary	Parathyroid gland Thyroid gland			Thymus	Posterior pituitary	Epiphysis	
Other	Central nervous system, Psyche	Mammary gland					Genitals Rectum, Anus	
Vertebra	H7, Bl-7, S1-2	B11-12, L1			H5-7, B2-4, L4-5	B8-10	L2-3, K3-S	
Tissue	Blood vessels	Connective tissue			Skin / Hair	Muscles / Tendons	Skeleton (Bones)	

2-1	2-2	2-3	2-4	2-5	2-6	2-7	2-8
							Kidney
Kidney / Bladder		Liver/ Bile	Lung / Large intstine		Spleen / Stomach		Heart / Small intestine
Frontal sinus Sphenoidal sinus		Sphenoidal sinus	Ethmoidal air cells		Maxillary sinus		Sine cavern
Pharyngeal tonsil		Palatine tonsil	Tubal tonsil		Laryngeal tonsils		Lingual tonsils
Ear (chin. 5 Elements)		Eye (back)	Nose / Smell		Tongue Taste		Inner ear
Epiphysis		Posterior pituitary	Thymus		Parathyroid gland Thyroid gland		Anterior pituitary
Genitals Rectum, Anus					Mammary gland		Central nervous system, Psyche
L2-3, K3-S		B8-10	H5-7, B2-4, L4-5		B11-12, L1		H7, BI-7, S1-2
Skeleton (Bones)		Muscels Tendons	Skin / Hair		Connective tissue		Blood vessels

Dental focus in the upper jaw	4-8	4-7	4-6	4-5	4-4	4-3	4-2	4-1
Relationship with the immune system	Adrenal gland Upper temporo-mandibular joint							
Organs	Heart / Small intestine	Ling/ Large intestin		Pancreas/ Stomach		Liver/ Bile	Kidney / Bladder	
Cranial cavities	Sine cavern	Ethmoidal air cells		Maxillary sinus		Sphenoidal sinus	Frontal sinus Sphenoidal sinus	
Tonsils	Lingual tonsile	Turbal tonsil		Laryngeal tonsils		Palatine tonsil	Pharyngeal tonsil	
Sensory organs	Outer and Middle ear	Nose Smell		Tongue/ Taste		Eye (front)	Ear (Chin. 5 Elements)	
Endocrine gland	"Energy budget" (Adrenal gland)			Mammary gland	Ovary	Testicle	Adrenal gland	
Other	Peripheral nervous system	Arteries	Veins	Lympha-tic vessels			Genitals Rectum, Anus	
Vertebra	H7, BI-7, S1-2	H5-7, B2-4 L4-5		B11-12, L1		B3-10	L2-3, K3-S	
Tissue	Blood vessels	Skin / Hair		Connective tissue		Muscles Tendons	Skeleton (Bones)	

3-1	3-2	3-3	3-4	3-5	3-6	3-7	3-8
Kidney / Bladder		Liver / Bile	Spleen / Stomach		Lung / Large intestine		Adrenal gland Upper temporo-mandibular joint Heart/ Small intestine
Frontal sinus Sphenoidal sinus		Maxillary sinus	Maxillary sinus		Ethmoidal air cells		Sine cavern
Pharyngeal tonsil		Palatine tonsil	Laryngeal tonsils		Tubal tonsil		Lingual tonsils
Ear (chin. 5 Elements)		Eye (front)	Tongue Taste		Nose / Smell		Outer and Middle ear
Adrenal gland		Ovary	Mammary gland Testicle				"Energy budget" (Adrenal gland)
Genitals Rectum, Anus			Lymphatic vessels		Arteries	Veins	Peripheral nervous system
L2-3, K3-S		B8-10	B11-12, L1		H5-7, B2-4, L4-5		H7, BI-7, S1-2
Skeleton (Bones)		Muscles Tendons	Connective tissue		Skin / Hair		Blood vessels

3.9.7 Metabolism

A derailed metabolism is a frequent cause of physical and mental complaints. If the metabolic processes within the body no longer run smoothly, the following problems may occur: pain, depression, irritability, disorders, digestive problems, poor concentration, exhaustion, burn-out and much more. Is important to recognize the causes within the metabolism through the appropriate diagnostics. For this purpose the clinical symptoms as well as laboratory findings are crucial. By supplementing the missing substances and via nutritional supplements, many things can be compensated in a gentle way.

A weak metabolism can be noticed especially in the mouth and teeth area. Gum diseases occur easier in a weaker body. If a immuno-deficiency is present, a tooth dies more readily.

3.9.7.1 Nutrition

„You are what you eat –
or what you have eaten"

Healthy eating and body cleansing can very quickly lead to an improved well being. There are diets, which can help to harmonise the metabolism and the hormones. What kind of food is beneficial for the individual person, depends on many different criteria. Via questionnaires and food diaries, one can see how a patient eats.

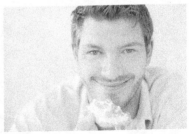

Fig. 72: Nutrition can help to harmonise the metabolism and dental health.

Considering the patient's illnesses and weaknesses one can individually work out what food is best for him or her. Tests can reveal food intolerances. They should be taken into account, when following a diet. These tests can also be done via EAV and kinesiology. Also the LTT test is suitable to show intolerances via blood tests.

3.9.7.2 Food supplements

EAV helps to establish what food supplements help the body to regenerate. They can then be administered specifically for a given amount of time. After an intervall of about three months, the levels should be checked afresh. Supplements can consist of vitamins, minerals, basica (substances to counteract an acidosis), natural remedies, enzymes, natural hormones and homeopathic medicines. If basica are given, the vitamin B 12 level should be checked and if needed complemented by subcutaneous injections. Vitamin B 12 can only be absorbed with a specific acidity of the stomach and this can be hampered by basica.

3.9.7.3 Detoxification

A long term absorption of environmental toxins, improper nutrition, or stress waste products, can cause a slagging of the tissue and a decreased responsiveness of the cells with its receptors and components within the cell. To cleanse the tissue, detoxification measures are recommended.

Fasting or a special diet can help detoxifications, homeopathic medicaments stimulate detoxification organs. The body detoxifies especially well via the feet. Recommended are foot baths with mustard, sage or electrolysis. Special Chinese herbal packs can be stuck to the sole of your feet in the evening to detoxify the body overnight. Specific vitamins and minerals also help a detoxification (for example, vitamin C, calcium and magnesium). Energetic methods like the bioresonance therapy are as well helpful in draining harmful substances and to detoxify. Especially after a dental treatment a detoxification might be advisable, since the body suffers due to medicaments and other substances.

3.9.7.4 Digestion

"In the intestine lurks death", is an old saying. Eating the wrong foods, lack of movement and stress leads to intestinal problems, like slagging or pollution of the intestine, a decreased capacity to absorb food, intolerances, increased permeability, decreased bowel movement, bloating, digestive problems or stomach pain.

Dentistry pays a lot of attention to the digestive system. The mouth is the start of the digestive system and intestinal problems are often the result in problems of the mucosa in the area of the mouth, such as periodontitis or bone deterioration. Important is the sanitation of the intestine via the right food, this can be helped with homeopathic treatments and also by restoring the intestinal flora. The bioresonance therapy has as also proven to be very successful. Movement is also very good for the intestine.

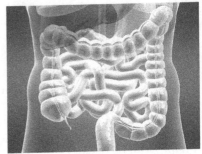

Abb. 73: A healty intestine means healthy gums.

3.9.7.5 Biohormones

„Everybody wants to live long but nobody wants to grow old", as Johann Nestroy said.

A loss of the hormonal balance is often the cause for illnesses or physical and mental disorders. The decisive factor is a sound knowledge of the hormonal correlations within the body. When diagnosing hormonal disturbances, the clinical symptoms caused by the lack of of hormones are recorded. A blood, saliva and urine test confirms the diagnosis. Slight disturbances can often be improved by lifestyle changes, an improved diet, cleaning measures and homeopathic treatments. If severe disturbances or fatigued glands are diagnosed, the missing hormones need to be supplemented. It is hereby crucial, that a hormone is given, that is identical to the human and that it is given in the right cyclical order.

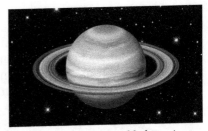

Fig. 74: A hormonal balance is important for the health in general and also for healthy teeth.

Anti Aging is not the pursuit for eternal youth, but attempting to age without or with less severe diseases.

3.9.8 Strong nerves

Due to our modern lifestyle, many patients have an irritated vegetative nervous system. We speak of bad nerves or nervousness. With holistic measures a regulation and harmonisation of the nerves can be achieved. Massages, vibration massages, biofeedback methods and the harmonisation of functional disturbances can herby be useful. Less stress on the jaw- and head joint can also result in relieving the autonomous nerves. This may result in an improvement of the cardiac arrhythmias, digestive problems, respiratory disorders and many more. The basic rhythm of the autonous nervous system might be improved.

3.9.8.1 Cranio-sacral therapy

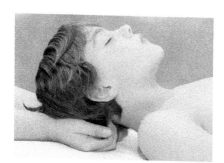

Fig. 75: Cranio-sacral therapy frees blockages.

Cranio-sacral therapy is a type of massage, which frees blockages in the skull, the spine and the sacrum, using very light touches.

The therapist is trying to find the rhythmical pulsations of the cerebrospinal fluid and tries to gently guide it. This can result in a better mobility within the craniosacral system. It also releases pressure from the nervous system. Blocked tissue in some areas can lead to orthopaedic distortions. Cranio-sacral therapy can help to free these blockages.

3.9.8.2   Biofeedback

With the help of a computer, biofeedback renders bodily functions visible, which are not normally noticed by the patient. This monitoring makes the patient aware of these functions.

Biofeedback works with a behavioural and theoretical learning approach: In realizing what is going wrong and subsequently learning to control bodily functions better. It can be used to improve the ability to relax. Also for rehabilitation and a better use of the masticator muscles, biofeedback is used. Biofeedback can be done with almost every bodily function. Especially common is the heart rate variability (HRV). Hereby the link between the heartbeat and breathing is measured, to establish the synergy between heart rhythm and breathing frequency. During training, the patient can learn to improve this and the whole nerve situation can benefit from it. It is also a good method to improve muscle relaxation. The relaxation is being shown on the computer and the patient then trains to relax the responsible muscles..

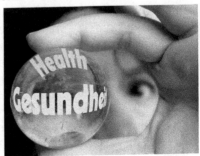

Fig. 76: Biofeedback helps to realize what is going wrong.

3.9.8.3   Bach flower therapy

According to Dr. Bach, any physical disease comes along with a mental imbalance. Bach flowers are supposed to re harmonise this imbalance. Via EAV or Kinesiology it can be tested, what kind of Bach flowers are best. There can then be administered against a fear of dentists or other problems.

3.9.8.4 Progressive muscle relaxation according to Jacobson

In progressive muscle relaxation according to Jacobson, the patient alters between tightening and relaxing the muscles. The aim is to learn the difference between relaxation and tension. This helps to relax and to better interconnect the muscle synapses. This is especially important in the area of the jaw muscles, since there is always an initial tension. Often, the patient does not even notice, when the chewing musculature is very tense.

3.9.8.5 Transcutaneous nerve stimulation (TENS)

TENS (transcutaneous nerve stimulation) helps to relax the masticatory muscles and the muscles of the neck. A device produces electric impulses which are transmitted to the relevant nerves via the skin. Impulses tension and relax the masticatory muscles without having to work. This relaxes the stressed nerve system of the masticatory muscles, and the pain is lessened. Furthermore, the muscles regain their ability to relax and to obtain their original length. This helps to have a more relaxed bite. The treatment and diagnosis is very good if the patient collaborates accordingly.

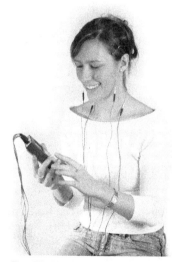

Fig. 77: Via transcutainious nerve stimulation (TENS) of the trigeminusnervs, which is responsible for the masticatory apparaturs the masticatory muscles are being relaxed.

3.9.8.6   Biostimulation by Nazarov

The biostimulation by Nazarov imitates the natural mechanical vibratory motion of the muscles. It can also be used on muscles which can no longer be tensioned. For this reason, it can be used for paralyzed muscles. The vibrations are transmitted to nerve, fascia and muscle tissue. This results in the tissue being cleaned and the transport of oxygen and minerals being improved. By purification of cell membranes and the exposure of ion channels, stimuli can be better transmitted.

3.9.8.7   Relaxation exercises

During our CMD-treatments, we try to develop relaxation methods, which are individually adapted for each patient. Regular exercises have to be done at home and then controlled and corrected in the praxis.

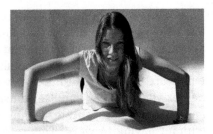

Fig. 78: Relaxation exercises should be individually adapted for each patient.

3.9.9 Good vibes

Every person, every body part and every illness has a vibe and a field. To get back to health, it is important to have the right vibes and the right field. This can be encouraged by different methods of the vibe and field therapy.

3.9.9.1   Homeopathy

Homeopathy is the treatment with homeopathic remedies.

A homeopathic agent is a tincture (for example Arnica tincture), diluted with water, alcohol or sugar (potentiated), this should be accompanied by a specific wave-like motion. The mother tincture

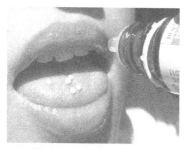

which is used causes a similar symptom as the disease to be treated. For example, the cinchona causes similar symptoms to malaria. If the quinine is potentiated homeopathically, these symptoms can be treated by stimulating the immune system.

Fig. 79: Homeopathy is a treatment applied in holistic dentistry.

3.9.9.2 Isopathy

Isopathy is a homeopathic therapy with isopathic substances. Hereby, one does not use substances that are similar to the disease, but the disease itself, homeopathically prepared. This stimulates the immune system to become active against this disease. For example, if a dental pulp inflammation is present, the tissue of the inflamed tooth nerve is used to extract the remedy.

3.9.9.3 Bioresonance therapy

Bioresonance therapy is a treatment which is done via two electrodes on the skin. They check out the resistance of the skin and function like an amplifier. It scans the vibrations of the body and changes them into better or different vibrations. Every illness or abnormal tissue is supposed to have a vibration, and inverted vibes can annihilate these bad vibrations and help a convalescence. The aim is to find the optimal vibration for the body.

3.9.9.4   Acupuncture

Acupuncture is a method in which fine needles are stuck into so called acupuncture points. Acupuncture points are fine points within the tissue which are verifiably more permeable and which allow a better contact with the autonomous nervous system. Via acupuncture points excess energy can be drained. Acupuncture is supposed to be helpful against pain and other chronic problems. In dentistry, acupuncture of the ear helps to relax the jaw muscles and it prevents the urge to gag. With the acupuncture of the mouth many problems can be cured.

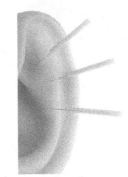

Fig. 80: Acupuncture helps to relax the autonomous nervous system.

3.9.9.5   Magnetic field therapy

The effect of the alternating magnetic field therapy is the improvement of the circulation and the cell metabolism. This is aimed to influence the metabolic processes of the cell membranes positively. Nerves should coordinate themselves better. I use magnetic field therapy for operations and dental treatments.

3.9.10 Posture

An upright posture is important to stay healthy and to have an attractive physical appearance. Science, which deals with posture, is dealing with this problem for a long time already. It is possible to have a healthy, elastic body even in old age.

Especially the bite or rather the malocclusion can be associated with a bad posture. Malfunctions in the jaw are always associated with the locomotory system. The bite is the posture of the mouth and the jaw. The jaw with its teeth, the jaw joint and the muscles are inseparably connected to the body via the skeleton, muscles, fascia and other anatomical structures throughout the whole body. Every change in the bite is an invasive intervention.

Patients with malocclusion have often orthopaedic problems. The cause for it is often not the bite but rather the orthopaedic problem which can cause problems with the bite. We call them rising problems or descending problems.

As part of the splint treatment, orthodontic treatments and bite improvements, it is useful to perform the following treatments within the realms of a posture therapy.

3.9.10.1 Posture – Functional Analysis

The bite is often the reason for many problems within the body. To establish the exact nature of the bite problems and the repercussions within the body, a good functional analysis is necessary. Herby we differentiate between a functional analysis with the focus on purely dentistry and a functional analysis which considers the whole body in relation to the bite.

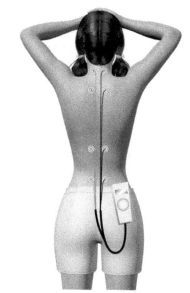

From the point of view of dentistry, we take the masticatory muscles into consideration, the position and the movement within the jaw joints, wrong bites and dental defects.

If we have a holistic approach to the bite, the posture of the spine, the muscle force, vegetative stress, the correlation with the sleep, and the stress, the feet are subject to.

Fig. 81: With a dynamic walk analysis one can analyse posture problems which are caused by the bite.

One assumes, that changes in the bite influence the whole body. The bite and the position of the teeth have a lot do with the body posture. Problems in the craniomandibular system might be related to a bad posture of the body.

Therefore it is very important to consider the posture when treating CMD. Pictures of the body are being taken. This is being repeated during the treatment to follow the course of the treatment. A better posture is being helped with bite improvements, posture exercises, osteopathy and foot treatments.

3.9.10.2 Posture Training

To obtain a better posture, certain rules are important. Regular exercises, as well as stretching exercises are crucial for a better success. Together with a bite improvement and stretching as well as the removal of blockages, a much better posture can be obtained. We monitor this via exercises, especially for CMD as well as behavioural training. 2-4 easy exercises are being chosen individual, they should be trained at home and then controlled in the praxis and corrected if necessary.

3.9.10.3 Feet

The feet are very important for the posture as well as for the situation within the craniomandibular area. There are different ways to improve the feet and their posture. One can work with neurologically effective foot orthotics (Podoorthesiology and Podoatiology), to activate certain muscle areas. Furthermore, the feet can be strengthened with foot gymnastic and other sport which invigorates the feet (cross country skiing, Nordic walking). Certain yoga exercises are also of interest as well as foot reflexology.

The End

This is not a scientific book but tries to put light into the dark of holistic dentistry. I tried to collect my experiences of 20 years. I have always tried to link conventional dentistry, as it is taught in academic medicine, with an holistic approach.

During many years of CMD treatments with chronic pain-, accident- and sleep apnoea patients, I found myself again and again facing new limits and new challenges. I started to open up more and more to so-called alternative methods. If nothing else helps and it serves the patient, it is the right way. In most cases the combination between conventional methods, which are recognized by academics and alternative methods which do no harm leads to success.

It is especially important to see the patient as an individual, to consider his/her history, individual problems and wishes and then to try to develop an adequate therapy. Some therapies take a long time. During these long term treatments, it is important to always consider the patient anew, to include possible changes into the therapy and if necessary to adapt or to change it.

Holistic dentistry is not the easiest way for a dentist, but it is definitely the most successful one I have ever tried. In holistic dentistry we work causally. That means we look for the underlying problems of a specific problem. If this cause is then eliminated, it can not cause other dental illnesses. This enables us to work on a long term scheme to prevent a loss of teeth and to keep the area of the mouth healthy. This should be the aim of the dentist and the patient.

In holistic dentistry the patient needs a lot of patience. Some problems cannot be made to disappear by magic but need a closer look and then a systematic treatment with the help of the patient. Only if you are ready it makes sense to engage in holistic dentistry.

„ The start is the most important part of the work."

(Platon)

Sources

Dr. Stefanie Morlok (the author): fig. 5, 15, 16, 20, 22, 26 a/b, 27 a/b/c, 29, 36, 51 (fig. to the right), 55, 58, 59, 60, 64, 70, 82

designbureauperstat / Dipl. Des. Arnold Perstat: fig. 3, 6, 7, 8, 10, 11, 12, 13, 14, 23, 24, 28, 31, 33, 35, 39, 40, 41, 42, 43, 44, 45, 46, 47, 48, 49, 50, 51 (fig. to the left), 52, 53, 54, 56, 62, 71, 81, all fig. on page 54 to 57, all fig. on page 106 to 109

Fotolia: fig. 1 (DN), fig. 4 (Andrea Danti), fig. 18 (DN) fig. 19 (DN); fig. 21 (contrastwerkstatt), fig. 25 a/b (Renate Maier), fig. 30 (Piumada-quila), fig. 32 (Héctor Manuel García), fig. 34 (Michael Tieck), fig. 37 (Paul Schwarzl), fig. 38 a/b/c (Christoph Hähnel), fig. 61 (Erwin Wodicka), fig. 66 (pressmaster), fig. 68 (contrastwerkstatt), fig. 69 (FFCucina Liz Collet), fig. 72 (detailblick), fig. 73 (Sebastian Kaulitzki), fig. 74 (Olga Sokolo), fig. 75 (Thomas Hammer), fig. 80 (Dirk Löffelbein)

Fotosearch: fig. 9

Shotshop: fig. 65 (Monkey Business)

schwa-medico GmbH: fig. 77

ResMed: fig. 63

pixelio.de: fig. 17 (Sabine Meyer), fig. 67 (Uwe Wagschal), fig. 76 (Sigrid Rossmann), fig. 78 (Stephanie Hofschlaeger), fig. 79 (Dr. Leonora Schwarz)

www.wikipedia.org: fig. 2

zebris Medical GmbH: fig. 57

ABOUT THE AUTHOR

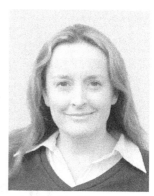

Dr. Stefanie Morlok is since 1994 practicing dentist in her praxis in Munich. Right from the start she tried to work with holistic methods and with an empathic approach in her praxis. A car crash and the resulting health problems lead her to carry out research and to study further to achieve an ideal and rounded treatment concept.

Fig. 82:
Dr. Stefanie Morlok

Her concern is the combination of scientifically proven, high quality Dentistry, with methods of holistic medicine, dentistry, and orthodontics. To mention are the test methods, the treatment with homeopathy and the vibration therapy. An important component in her treatment concept are improper strains of the jaw and it's repercussions on the rest of the body. She treats according to the classical bionator therapy of Balters.

The collaboration with competent therapist and a tight contact with them is a fundamental part of her concept. Anthroposophic aspects of medicine and dentistry are part of her practice. She combines dentistry, dental surgery and orthodontics in one surgery.

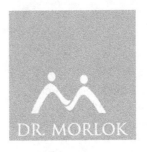

Dr. Stefanie Morlok
MSc Orthodontics, Dentist

Holistic Dentistry
Specialist treatment centre for CMD, Jaw disorders and
diseases, dental treatment of sleep disturbances

Our therapeutic specialisation:
Holistic dentistry, CMD – craniomandibular dysfunction,
dental splints, snoring splints,
Holistic Orthodontics

The Praxis Dr. Morlok is one of the few practises Europe wide, which specialises in the treatment of CMD. Our treatment of craniomandibular dysfunction and our dental care are carried out to the highest standards. Our team focuses on an excellent training as well as an ongoing quality control through our introduced quality management. Our staff undertakes continual training to remain up to date with current practises. With us your dental care is always in good hands.

Dr. Stefanie Morlok
Zur Aussichtswarte 15, 86919 Utting, Tel: 0049 (08806) 958630

www.drmorlok.com

CPSIA information can be obtained
at www.ICGtesting.com
Printed in the USA
BVHW040154190220
572794BV00010B/90

9 783981 850802